Device-Based Arrhythmia Monitoring

Editors

SUNEET MITTAL
DAVID J. SLOTWINER

CARDIAC ELECTROPHYSIOLOGY CLINICS

www.cardiacEP.theclinics.com

Consulting Editors
RANJAN K. THAKUR
ANDREA NATALE

September 2021 • Volume 13 • Number 3

ELSEVIER

1600 John F. Kennedy Boulevard • Suite 1800 • Philadelphia, Pennsylvania, 19103-2899

http://www.theclinics.com

CARDIAC ELECTROPHYSIOLOGY CLINICS Volume 13, Number 3
September 2021 ISSN 1877-9182, ISBN-13: 978-0-323-89722-8

Editor: Joanna Collett
Developmental Editor: Hannah Almira Lopez

Cardiac Electrophysiology Clinics (ISSN 1877-9182) is published quarterly by Elsevier Inc., 360 Park Avenue South, New York, NY 10010-1710. Months of issue are March, June, September, and December. Subscription prices are $238.00 per year for US individuals, $502.00 per year for US institutions, $249.00 per year for Canadian individuals, $535.00 per year for Canadian institutions, $303.00 per year for international individuals, $535.00 per year for international institutions and $100.00 per year for US, Canadian and international students/residents. To receive student/resident rate, orders must be accompanied by name of affiliated institution, date of term, and the signature of program/residency coordinator on institution letterhead. Orders will be billed at individual rate until proof of status is received. Foreign air speed delivery is included in all Clinics subscription prices. All prices are subject to change without notice. **POSTMASTER:** Send address changes to Cardiac Electrophysiology Clinics, Elsevier Health Sciences Division, Subscription Customer Service, 3251 Riverport Lane, Maryland Heights, MO 63043. **Customer Service: 1-800-654-2452 (US and Canada). From outside of the US and Canada, call 314-477-8871. Fax: 314-447-8029. E-mail: JournalsCustomerService-usa@elsevier.com (for print support); JournalsOnlineSupport-usa@elsevier.com (for online support).**

Reprints. For copies of 100 or more of articles in this publication, please contact the Commercial Reprints Department, Elsevier Inc., 360 Park Avenue South, New York, NY 10010-1710. Tel.: 212-633-3874; Fax: 212-633-3820; E-mail: reprints@elsevier.com.

Cardiac Electrophysiology Clinics is covered in *MEDLINE/PubMed (Index Medicus)*.

Contributors

CONSULTING EDITORS

RANJAN K. THAKUR, MD, MPH, MBA, FHRS
Professor of Medicine and Director, Arrhythmia
Service, Thoracic and Cardiovascular Institute,
Sparrow Health System, Michigan State
University, Lansing, Michigan, USA

ANDREA NATALE, MD, FACC, FHRS
Executive Medical Director of the Texas
Cardiac Arrhythmia Institute, St. David's
Medical Center, Professor, Dell Medical
School, University of Texas at Austin, Austin,
Texas, USA; National Medical Director,
Cardiac Electrophysiology, Consulting
Professor, Division of Cardiology, Stanford
University, Stanford, California, USA; Clinical
Professor of Medicine, Case Western Reserve
University, Cleveland, Ohio, USA; Director,
Interventional Electrophysiology, Scripps
Clinic, San Diego, California, USA

EDITORS

SUNEET MITTAL, MD, FACC, FHRS
Department of Cardiology, Snyder Center for
Comprehensive Atrial Fibrillation, Valley Health
System, Ridgewood, New Jersey, USA;
Director, Electrophysiology, Valley Health
System, Paramus, New Jersey, USA

DAVID J. SLOTWINER, MD, FACC, FHRS
Chief, Division of Cardiology, NewYork-
Presbyterian Queens, Assistant Professor of
Medicine, School of Population Health
Sciences, Weill Cornell Medicine, New York,
New York, USA

AUTHORS

RYAN AHMED, MS
User Experience Research Specialist II, Health
Services and Informatics Research, Parkview
Mirro Center for Research and Innovation, Fort
Wayne, Indiana, USA

TINA ALLMANDINGER, BSN, RN
Supervisor, Arrhythmia Diagnostic Center,
Parkview Physicians Group, Fort Wayne,
Indiana, USA

**ADRIAN BARANCHUK, MD, FACC, FRCPC,
FCCS, FSIAC**
Department of Cardiac Electrophysiology and
Pacing, Professor of Medicine, Department of
Cardiology, Kingston General Hospital,
Queen's University, Kingston, Ontario, Canada

SILVIA CASTELLETTI, MD
Istituto Auxologico Italiano, IRCCS – Center for
Cardiac Arrhythmias of Genetic Origin, Milan,
Italy

CARLY DALEY, MS
Research Scientist, Health Services and
Informatics Research, Parkview Mirro Center
for Research and Innovation, Fort Wayne,
Indiana, USA

JEROEN DAUW, MD
Doctoral School of Medicine and Life Sciences,
Hasselt University, Hasselt, Belgium;
Cardiology Department, Ziekenhuis Oost-
Limburg, Genk, Belgium

SÉBASTIEN DEFERM, MD
Doctoral School of Medicine and Life Sciences, Hasselt University, Hasselt, Belgium; Cardiology Department, Ziekenhuis Oost-Limburg, Genk, Belgium

STIJN EVENS, MSc
Qompium NV, Hasselt, Belgium

PAUL A. FRIEDMAN, MD
Professor of Medicine, Department of Cardiovascular Medicine, Mayo Clinic, Rochester, Minnesota, USA

HENRI GRUWEZ, MD
Department of Cardiovascular Sciences, KU Leuven, Cardiology, University Hospitals Leuven, Leuven, Belgium; Doctoral School of Medicine and Life Sciences, Hasselt University, Hasselt, Belgium; Cardiology Department, Ziekenhuis Oost-Limburg, Genk, Belgium

PETER HAEMERS, MD, PhD
Department of Cardiovascular Sciences, KU Leuven, Cardiology, University Hospitals Leuven, Leuven, Belgium

KENNETH P. HOYME, MSEE
Senior Fellow, Global Product Cybersecurity, Boston Scientific, St Paul, Minnesota, USA

CHARLES J. LOVE, MD
Professor of Medicine, Director, Cardiac Rhythm Device Services, Johns Hopkins School of Medicine and Hospital, Baltimore, Maryland, USA

RUTH MASTERSON CREBER, PhD, MSc, RN
Associate Professor of Population Health Sciences, Division of Health Informatics, Weill Cornell Medicine, New York, New York, USA

MICHAEL MIRRO, MD, FACC, FHRS, FAHA, FACP
Senior VP, Parkview Health System, Chief Academic Research Officer, Parkview Mirro Center for Research and Innovation, Fort Wayne, Indiana, USA

SUNEET MITTAL, MD, FACC, FHRS
Department of Cardiology, Snyder Center for Comprehensive Atrial Fibrillation, Valley Health System, Ridgewood, New Jersey, USA; Director, Electrophysiology, Valley Health System, Paramus, New Jersey, USA

ROD S. PASSMAN, MD, MSCE
Jules J. Reingold Professor of Electrophysiology, Professor of Medicine and Preventive Medicine, Department of Internal Medicine, Division of Cardiology, Northwestern University Feinberg School of Medicine, Chicago, Illinois, USA

LAURENT PISON, MD, PhD
Cardiology Department, Ziekenhuis Oost-Limburg, Genk, Belgium

TINE PROESMANS, MSc
Qompium NV, Hasselt, Belgium

JOHN RICKARD, MD, MPH
Staff Physician, Department of Cardiovascular Medicine, Section of Cardiac Electrophysiology, Heart, Vascular, and Thoracic Institute, Cleveland Clinic, Cleveland, Ohio, USA

DAVID J. SANDERS, MD
General Cardiology Fellow, Department of Internal Medicine, Division of Cardiology, Rush University, Chicago, Illinois, USA

PETER J. SCHWARTZ, MD
Istituto Auxologico Italiano, IRCCS – Center for Cardiac Arrhythmias of Genetic Origin, Milan, Italy

GERALD A. SERWER, MD
Professor of Pediatrics, University of Michigan, UM Congenital Heart Center, Michigan Medicine, Ann Arbor, Michigan, USA

ARJUN N. SHARMA, BSc, MD
Resident Physician, Internal Medicine, Department of Medicine, Kingston General Hospital, Queen's University, Kingston, Ontario, Canada

SUDAR SHIELDS, MSEE
Product Security Systems Architect, Global Product Cybersecurity, Boston Scientific, St Paul, Minnesota, USA

KONSTANTINOS C. SIONTIS, MD
Assistant Professor of Medicine, Department of Cardiovascular Medicine, Mayo Clinic, Rochester, Minnesota, USA

DAVID J. SLOTWINER, MD, FACC, FHRS
Chief, Division of Cardiology, NewYork-Presbyterian Queens, Assistant Professor of Medicine, School of Population Health Sciences, Weill Cornell Medicine, New York, New York, USA

TAMMY TOSCOS, PhD
Research Scientist and Director, Health Services and Informatics Research, Parkview Mirro Center for Research and Innovation, Fort Wayne, Indiana, USA

MEGHAN READING TURCHIOE, PhD, MPH, RN
Instructor of Population Health Sciences, Division of Health Informatics, Weill Cornell Medicine, New York, New York, USA

PIETER VANDERVOORT, MD, PhD
Doctoral School of Medicine and Life Sciences, Hasselt University, Hasselt, Belgium; Cardiology Department, Ziekenhuis Oost-Limburg, Genk, Belgium

FREDERIK H. VERBRUGGE, MD, PhD
Centre for Cardiovascular Diseases, University Hospital Brussels, Jette, Belgium; Faculty of Medicine and Pharmacy, Vrije Universiteit

Brussel, Brussels, Belgium; Biomedical Research Institute, Faculty of Medicine and Life Sciences, Hasselt University, Hasselt, Belgium

SHAUNA WAGNER, BSN, RN
Research Project Leader II, Health Services and Informatics Research, Parkview Mirro Center for Research and Innovation, Fort Wayne, Indiana, USA

JEREMIAH WASSERLAUF, MD, MS
Assistant Professor of Medicine, Cardiac Electrophysiology, Department of Internal Medicine, Division of Cardiology, Rush University, Chicago, Illinois, USA

RIK WILLEMS, MD, PhD
Department of Cardiovascular Sciences, KU Leuven, Cardiology, University Hospitals Leuven, Leuven, Belgium

BRYAN WILNER, MD
Fellow, Department of Cardiovascular Medicine, Section of Cardiac Electrophysiology, Heart, Vascular, and Thoracic Institute, Cleveland Clinic, Cleveland, Ohio, USA

BO GREGERS WINKEL, MD, PhD
University Hospital Copenhagen, Rigshospitalet, Department of Cardiology, Copenhagen, Denmark

Contents

Ambulatory external electrocardiography (AECG) monitoring is effective as an evidence-based diagnostic tool when suspicion for cardiac arrhythmia is high. Multiple modalities of AECG monitoring exist, with unique advantages and limitations that predict effectiveness in a variety of clinical settings. Knowledge of these characteristics allows appropriate use of AECG, maximizing patient adherence, diagnostic yield, and cost-effectiveness. In addition, new technology has allowed the development of a modern generation of devices that offer increased efficacy and functionality compared with Holter monitors.

The implantable loop recorder (ILR) is a subcutaneous, single-lead, electrocardiographic (ECG) monitoring device used for diagnosis in patients with recurrent, unexplained episodes of palpitations or syncope, for long-term monitoring in patients at risk for atrial fibrillation (AF), and to guide clinical management in patients with known AF. These devices are capable of storing and transmitting ECG data automatically in response to a significant bradyarrhythmia or tachyarrhythmia or in response to patient activation. This document aims to review the clinical utility of ILRs for arrhythmia monitoring in common clinical situations such as syncope, cryptogenic stroke, and management of patients with known AF.

Remote monitoring of permanent pacemakers and implantable cardiac defibrillators has undergone considerable advances over the past several decades. Advancement of technology has created the ability for remote monitoring of implantable cardiac devices; a device can monitor its own function, record arrhythmias, and transmit data to health care providers without frequent in-office checks, shown to be as safe as in-office interrogation. Remote monitoring allows earlier detection of clinically actionable events, reduces incidence of inappropriate shocks, and allows earlier detection of atrial fibrillation. App-based remote monitoring provides patients with rapid access to their cardiac data, which may improve compliance with remote monitoring.

> Guidelines exist for monitoring to diagnose and manage patients with several different conditions. Although there have been recent updates to the guidelines, the constantly evolving and advancing nature of the technologies creates a gap at times between the newest monitors, the indications for their use, and the reimbursement by the payers. The key element to the choice of the modality of monitoring remains matching the correct technology to the type, severity, frequency, and duration of the patient's symptoms.

> Movement of information from a cardiac implantable electronic device to an electronic health record (EHR) can be a complex and multistep process. It requires unambiguous patient identification, device identification, standardized semantic and syntactic data nomenclature, common secure data transfer methodology, and structured reporting within the EHR. Common workflow using a commonly accepted methodology, such as the implantable device cardiac observation profile or protocol, is mandatory. Once information reaches the EHR, a uniform report structure appropriate for the consumer (physician or patient) is needed. Often there may be separate reports for each consumer class. Finally, patient acceptance and consent are required.

> This review provides an overview of the literature on the organization, staffing, and structure of remote monitoring (RM) clinics, primarily from countries in Western Europe and United States, as well as the challenges, considerations, and future directions for RM clinic models of care. Using a current case example of an RM clinic in the Midwestern United States, this document provides key information from the viewpoint of a clinic undergoing a shift in workflow. Finally, this review distills key considerations for RM management for electrophysiology clinics, vendors and industry, and policy makers.

> The ability to remotely reprogram a cardiac implantable electronic device (CIED) and the ability to remotely install software or firmware updates would reduce the need for in-office visits and could provide a mechanism to rapidly deploy important software or firmware updates. The challenges of implementing remote reprogramming of cardiac implantable electronic devices are no longer technical. Using asymmetric cryptography, sophisticated end-to-end secure communication protocols and hardware accelerators, the resources required to identify and take advantage of a cybersecurity vulnerability of a single CIED would be very significant and likely well beyond the gain that an intruder would deem worthwhile.

algorithmic analysis for rhythm determination to more complex deep machine learning methods that have led to the realization of fully automated humanlike rhythm determination in real-time.

Spurred by federal legislation, professional organizations, and patients themselves, patient access to data from electronic cardiac devices is increasingly transparent. Patients can collect data through consumer devices and access data traditionally shared only with health care providers. These data may improve screening, self-management, and shared decision-making for cardiac arrhythmias, but challenges remain, including patient comprehension, communication with providers, and sustained engagement. Ways to address these challenges include leveraging visualizations that support comprehension, involving patients in designing and developing patient-facing digital tools, and establishing clear practices and goals for data exchange with health care providers.

CARDIAC ELECTROPHYSIOLOGY CLINICS

SERIES OF RELATED INTEREST

Cardiology Clinics
Available at: https://www.cardiology.theclinics.com/
Heart Failure Clinics
Available at: https://www.heartfailure.theclinics.com/
Interventional Cardiology Clinics
Available at: https://www.interventional.theclinics.com/

THE CLINICS ARE AVAILABLE ONLINE!
Access your subscription at:
www.theclinics.com

Foreword
Device-Based Arrhythmia Monitoring

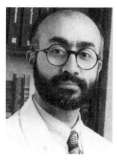
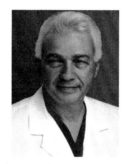

Ranjan K. Thakur, MD, MPH, MBA, FHRS   Andrea Natale, MD, FACC, FHRS

Editors

We are pleased to welcome Drs Mittal and Slotwiner as coeditors of this issue of the *Cardiac Electrophysiology Clinics* devoted to the advances in Device-Based Arrhythmia Monitoring.

Arrhythmia monitoring started with the advent of the ambulatory 24-hour Holter monitoring and then advanced to longer-term (30 days) monitoring. Advances in technology enabled cardiac implantable electronic device (pacemaker and defibrillator)-based arrhythmia surveillance and the implantable loop recorder, originally envisioned for diagnosis of unexplained syncope, but indications quickly expanded to include suspected arrhythmias and cryptogenic stroke to look for paroxysmal atrial fibrillation.

While technological advances have been tremendous, by enabling these developments, we are at an inflection point in technological innovation fueled by development of 5-G and artificial intelligence. The future is bright and limited only by imagination. Future developments will expand technology-assisted diagnostic prowess, expand remote device programming, and increase patient convenience, as the new generation of tech-savvy patients will demand it and change workflows in our clinics. Wearable cardiac and arrhythmia monitors will have an impact on diagnosis and monitoring of arrhythmias. Many of these technological developments are too recent to ascertain what role it may have and how they may be utilized. Many of

these advances will have to be balanced with the challenges posed by cybersecurity and legal issues.

Drs Mittal and Slotwiner have assembled a group of experts from academia and industry who have a focus on these issues of arrhythmia monitoring, and the articles in this issue of the *Cardiac Electrophysiology Clinics* will update the readers on the developments in this field, contemporary issues, and what the future may hold. We congratulate them for a unique summary of these issues in arrhythmia monitoring.

Ranjan K. Thakur, MD, MPH, MBA, FHRS
Sparrow Thoracic and Cardiovascular Institute
Michigan State University
1440 East Michigan Avenue; Suite 400
Lansing, MI 48912, USA

Andrea Natale, MD, FACC, FHRS
Texas Cardiac Arrhythmia Institute
Center for Atrial Fibrillation at
St. David's Medical Center
1015 East 32nd Street, Suite 516
Austin, TX 78705, USA

E-mail addresses:
thakur@msu.edu (R.K. Thakur)
andrea.natale@stdavids.com (A. Natale)

Card Electrophysiol Clin 13 (2021) xiii
https://doi.org/10.1016/j.ccep.2021.06.002
1877-9182/21/© 2021 Published by Elsevier Inc.

cardiacEP.theclinics.com

Preface
Device-Based Arrhythmia Monitoring

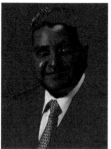   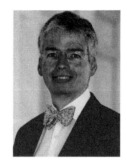

Suneet Mittal, MD, FACC, FHRS   David J. Slotwiner, MD, FACC, FHRS
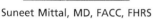
Editors

The transformation of device-based arrhythmia monitoring since the release of the first Holter monitor in 1962 reflects the broader trajectory of how advancements in technology, scientific evidence, and patient/consumer preferences are changing the way health care is delivered. The technological feat of being able to record 24 hours of heart rhythm tracings in a pocket-sized device was made possible, in large part, by the newly developed transistor. Today, thanks to countless technological innovations, medical advancements in the treatment of arrhythmias, and the desire of individuals to have agency over their health care, the estimated 3.6 billion people who have smartphones can download a free app that, using the device's flashlight, can obtain a surrogate marker for a single-lead electrocardiogram.[1] Device-based heart rhythm monitoring is now widely available not only to patients but also the general public. The data are used to manage disease as well as to maintain health. Devices range from diagnostic to life-sustaining. Scientific endeavors to help guide use of these devices continue to grow, as do the challenges of managing the data that they produce.

In this issue of *Cardiac Electrophysiology Clinics*, we provide an overview of the state-of-the-art of device-based arrhythmia monitoring. We begin with medical grade arrhythmia monitoring devices that now extend the diagnostic power of wearable devices and provide the option of telemetry, catering to a broad range of clinical scenarios. Implantable loop recorders extend the diagnostic power even further and have become critical diagnostic tools for patients with cryptogenic stroke or syncope. Next, we turn to remote monitoring of implantable cardiac rhythm management devices. A large body of evidence now exists supporting remote monitoring as standard of care for these patients, which has been incorporated into clinical practice guidelines. Yet organizing remote monitoring centers and managing the volume of data remain a tremendous challenge, which we address as well. The threat of cybersecurity breaches is ever present in our modern world, yet the ability to remotely monitor and potentially reprogram implantable pacemakers and defibrillators could provide significant benefits for many patients around the world, particularly those living in remote regions. We review the present security measures

Card Electrophysiol Clin 13 (2021) xv–xvi
https://doi.org/10.1016/j.ccep.2021.06.001
1877-9182/21/© 2021 Published by Elsevier Inc.

in place and explain why remote reprogramming, with the proper clinical guardrails, is very secure and unlikely to be a target of cybersecurity hackers.

Three articles in this issue are devoted to digital health tools for arrhythmia detection and management. Smartphones and other consumer wearables are democratizing the ability of individuals to record their heart rhythm, screen for atrial fibrillation, and monitor for potential proarrhythmia via QT interval monitoring. Looking into the future, we see how artificial intelligence is emerging as a powerful tool in arrhythmia monitoring and is likely to become an important clinical tool. We conclude by closing the loop and providing patients with direct access to their data, looking at the opportunity this has for empowering patients as well as the challenge it poses for providing the data in a meaningful and useful format for the diverse public.

When Norman Holter introduced the first prototype of his monitor in 1947 weighing over 36 kgs and worn as a backpack, it is doubtful he would have predicted the field today. Similarly, it is difficult for us to imagine what the field will look like in 65 years. But what is unlikely to change is the need for monitoring the heart rhythm and treating arrhythmias. The progress we have made has been possible thanks to the pioneers before us. We hope others will extend the knowledge and experience summarized in these articles and continue this innovation.

Suneet Mittal, MD, FACC, FHRS
Electrophysiology
Valley Health System
970 Linwood Avenue
Paramus, NJ 07652, USA

David J. Slotwiner, MD, FACC, FHRS
Division of Cardiology
New York Presbyterian Queens
56-45 Main Street
Flushing, NY 11355, USA

School of Population Health Sciences
Weill Cornell Medicine
1300 York Ave
New York, NY 11065, USA

E-mail addresses:
mittsu@valleyhealth.com (S. Mittal)
djs2001@med.cornell.edu (D.J. Slotwiner)

REFERENCE

1. At the Heart of the Invention: Development of the Holter Monitor. Available at: https://si-siris.blogspot.com/2011/10/at-heart-of-invention-development-of.html. Accessed May 16, 2021.

Ambulatory External Electrocardiography Monitoring: Holter, Extended Holter, Mobile Cardiac Telemetry Monitoring

Arjun N. Sharma, BSc, MD[a],
Adrian Baranchuk, MD, FACC, FRCPC, FCCS, FSIAC[b,c],*

KEYWORDS

- Holter • Device • Telemetry • Ambulatory • ECG

KEY POINTS

- Ambulatory external electrocardiography (AECG) monitoring is effective at diagnosing arrhythmia in patients presenting with palpitations, syncope, or presyncope.
- External AECG monitoring has additional utility in the monitoring of patients following pharmacologic, device-based, or invasive therapy for arrhythmia.
- Diagnostic yield of external loop monitors and mobile cardiac telemetry systems exceeds Holter and event recorders in the investigation of palpitations, presyncope, and syncope.
- Device selection and monitoring duration should be chosen based on clinical characteristics of the arrhythmia suspected to be causing the patient's symptoms.

INTRODUCTION

Background

Ambulatory external electrocardiography (AECG) monitors have a wide variety of clinical applications in diagnosis and treatment of arrhythmias. AECG has long been used to evaluate patients presenting with shortness of breath, chest pain, palpitations, or syncope in the outpatient setting.[1] AECG also has use in evaluating efficacy of prescribed antiarrhythmic treatment, assessing burden of arrhythmia, and in diagnosis of asymptomatic arrhythmias.[1,2]

The original mobile radioelectrocardiogram was taken by Norman Jefferis Holter in the late 1940s following the development of electrocardiography for clinical use in the early twentieth century.[3] Developments in electrode, wireless connectivity, and battery technology facilitated the evolution of multiple AECG modalities, each with unique advantages and disadvantages.[2,4] Multiple modalities of AECG monitors now exist: continuous (Holter-type) monitors, event monitors, external loop recorders (ELRs), and mobile cardiac telemetry (MCT). General characteristics of each modality are summarized in **Table 1**.

Holter Monitors

Continuous Holter monitors are portable multichannel devices designed to be worn by the patient in an uninterrupted fashion over a

[a] Internal Medicine, Department of Medicine, Kingston General Hospital, Queen's University, 76 Stuart Street, Kingston, Ontario K7L 2V7, Canada; [b] Department of Cardiac Electrophysiology and Pacing, Kingston General Hospital, Kingston, Ontario, Canada; [c] Department of Cardiology, Kingston General Hospital, Queen's University, 76 Stuart Street, Kingston, Ontario K7L 2V7, Canada
* Corresponding author. Department of Cardiology, Kingston General Hospital, Queen's University, 76 Stuart Street, Kingston, Ontario K7L 2V7, Canada.
E-mail address: adrian.baranchuk@kingstonhsc.ca

Card Electrophysiol Clin 13 (2021) 427–438
https://doi.org/10.1016/j.ccep.2021.04.003

Table 1
Review of external ambulatory external electrocardiography modalities

Monitor Type	Monitoring Duration (d)	Recording Type	Event Triggers	Leads	Real-time Monitoring	Advantages	Limitations
Holter	≤14[a]	Continuous	NA	3–12	No	Quantitative analysis of arrhythmia; 12-lead recording; Holter parameters	Patient noncompliance with increasing duration of monitoring
Patch	≤14	Continuous	NA	1–2	No	Ease of use; high adherence; self-contained leads; waterproof	Signal quality variation with body type; lack of multilead recording
Event	≤14	Event	Manual	1	No	High degree of symptom-rhythm correlation	Unable to capture asymptomatic or incapacitating arrhythmia
ELR	≤30	Event	Manual, automatic[a]	1–3	No	High diagnostic yield; capture of arrhythmic onset	Requires continuous use of the device throughout the monitoring period
MCT	≤30	Continuous, event	Manual, automatic	1–3	Yes	High diagnostic yield; immediate alarm generation; real-time monitoring	May be bulky or uncomfortable; resource intensive; not widely available

Choice of AECG modality should be dictated by patient factors such as expected adherence in addition to the clinical factors summarized here. Characteristics and features of each modality may differ between devices. The sequential use of multiple AECG modalities may be useful in improving overall diagnostic yield while preserving cost-effectiveness.

Abbreviation: NA, not available.
[a] May not be available in all devices.

predetermined period.[1] The term extended Holter has no strict or unanimous definition but may refer to use of a Holter monitor beyond 24 or 48 hours, and up to 14 days with certain devices. Following the recording period, devices are returned to a central location where data are analyzed.[1] Analysis includes a combination of automated and technician interpretation, the summary of which is delivered to the referring care provider.[4]

Holter monitors are available in 2-lead, 3-lead, or 12-lead configurations. Continuous multilead recording may allow the diagnosis of specific arrhythmic causes (**Fig. 1**) or subtle electrocardiographic mechanisms of arrhythmia (**Fig. 2**), or the avoidance of unnecessary intervention (**Fig. 3**).[5–7] Holter reports are often semistandardized, with multiple parameters and commonly reported analyses included.[4] These analyses, including heart rate turbulence (HRT), heart rate variability (HRV), premature ventricular contraction (PVC) burden, and systolic pauses, have clinical and research value and are expanded on later.

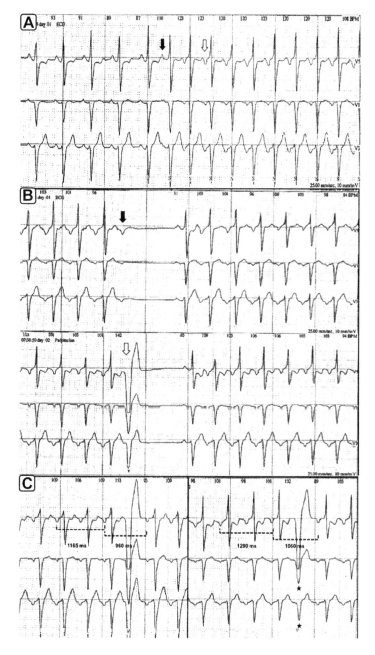

Fig. 1. A 55-year-old man presented with a long history of palpitations. A 24-hour Holter monitor revealed a regular narrow-complex tachycardia starting with a PAC (*A, black arrow*) with evident R-P>P-R (*A, white arrow*). A long-RP tachycardia was identified, suggesting a differential diagnosis of atrial tachycardia (AT), orthodromic atrioventricular (AV) reentrant tachycardia, and atypical AV-nodal reentrant tachycardia. The tachycardia spontaneously terminated with a nonpremature P wave (*B, black arrow*). Another episode of termination occurred with a premature ventricular contraction (PVC) not conducted to the atrium (*B, white arrow*), excluding a diagnosis of AT. Observed PVCs were found to advance atrial activation during His-refractory periods without termination of the tachycardia (*C*), suggesting the presence of an AV accessory pathway. An accessory pathway was later identified and ablated. (*Adapted from* Enriquez et al.; with permission.[5])

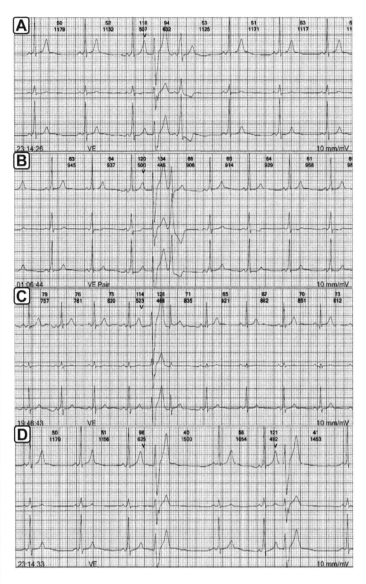

Fig. 2. A 21-year-old man presented with a history of palpitations. A 12-lead electrocardiogram (ECG) showed minimal ventricular preexcitation. A 24-hour Holter monitor was used and showed spontaneous monomorphic PVCs with varying degrees of postectopic ventricular preexcitation. The variation in QRS morphology can be explained by PVC coupling interval-dependent retrograde penetration of the AV node, accessory pathway, or both. Maximal preexcitation (coupling intervals of 507 and 500 milliseconds) was facilitated by retrograde penetration of the AV node (*A, B*) leading to preferential anterograde conduction through the accessory pathway. Retrograde penetration of the accessory pathway (coupling interval of 523 milliseconds) produced a postectopic QRS complex without preexcitation (*C*). Retrograde penetration of both pathways (coupling interval of 625 milliseconds) produced a complete block of the postectopic beat (*D*). (*Adapted from* Longo and Baranchuk; with permission.[6])

However, reporting of symptoms and adherence to 24-hour monitoring systems is often poor despite adequate patient education.[1] Furthermore, Holter devices can be bulky or uncomfortable and must be removed for showering or bathing. These limitations and the short duration of standard Holter monitoring may explain its poor diagnostic yield, estimated to be only 10% to 15% for palpitations and 1% to 5% for syncope and atrial fibrillation (AF) after cryptogenic stroke.[1,8,9] Common indications for Holter monitoring and its expected diagnostic yield are summarized in **Table 2**.

With these limitations in mind, a new generation of continuous monitoring devices (so-called patch monitors) were developed to be applied as a single unit adhesively to the chest.[10] These devices are used for 7 to 14 days but are limited to 1-lead or 2-lead recordings and may suffer from signal distortion with differing body morphologies.[1,11]

The frequency of suspected arrhythmias is often the most important factor in determining the length and modality of AECG monitoring. In many settings, the diagnostic yield of AECG increases proportional to duration of monitoring.[8,10,12–16] An extended duration of monitoring may be achieved with the use of longer-term Holter monitors, or with the use of other modalities.[9,17]

Event Recorders

Event recorders are small devices carried by patients for up to 30 days and activated at the time of symptom onset. They capture a short (30–

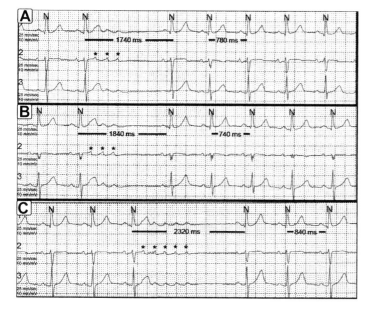

Fig. 3. A 67-year-old man was assessed for routine follow-up after pulmonary vein isolation for paroxysmal atrial fibrillation, including 24-hour Holter monitoring. Review of patient history and recordings identified multiple asymptomatic pauses of varying lengths (A–C). Each pause included a nonsustained and nonconducted AT with P wave morphology differing from the sinus rhythm. The AT, possibly originating from the pulmonary vein isolation ablation scar, causes overdrive suppression of the sinus node and concealed antegrade penetration of the AV node, leading to sinus pause and AV node conduction failure. Proper recognition and interpretation of these physiologic and benign mechanisms through AECG monitoring avoided unneeded intervention. (*Adapted from* Diez et al.; with permission.[7])

180 seconds), single-lead electrocardiogram (ECG), which is then transmitted via telephone to a central monitoring station for interpretation and analysis.[1] Event recorders offer symptom-rhythm correlation superior to Holter monitors in patients presenting with palpitations, presyncope, or other symptoms suggestive of cardiac arrhythmia.[18,19] In 1 randomized study of patients presenting with palpitations, capture of symptomatic arrhythmia was made in 119 patients with event recorders compared with 74 patients with Holter monitors (P<.01).[20] In addition, total cost of monitoring was smaller in the event recorder group. Indications for event recorder use are summarized in **Table 2**.

Despite their advantages, event recorders do not capture asymptomatic arrhythmia, and are not applicable in the investigation of incapacitating symptoms such as nonprodromal syncope.[21] Even with successful identification of arrhythmia, the lack of looping or continuous recording prevents observation of arrhythmic initiation and quantification of arrhythmic burden. Although event recorders still remain in use, it is probable that this technology will become obsolete as ELR and MCT devices become cheaper and more widely available.

External Loop Recorders

ELRs are multilead devices used for up to 30 days at a time. ELRs continuously record ECG data but do not store all recordings in long-term memory; instead, segments (loops) are committed to short-term memory and constantly deleted as recording continues. When the device is triggered,

Table 2					
Ambulatory external electrocardiography indications and estimated diagnostic yield					
Indication	Holter (%)	Patch (%)	Event (%)	ELR (%)	MCT (%)
Palpitations	10–15	50–70	50–60	70–85	70–85
Syncope	1–5	5–10	NA[a]	15–25	15–25
Stroke (AF)	1–10	5–10	NA[a]	2–20	5–25
Chest pain (CAD)	Poor (diagnosis) unclear (prognosis)	Not studied	Not studied	Not studied	Not studied

Estimated diagnostic yields and overall utility are based on summarized data from multiple studies, systematic reviews, and meta-analyses.[1,8,15–17,22,23,25,29,37,38,40–42]

Abbreviation: CAD, coronary artery disease.

[a] Patient-triggered devices should not be used in the investigation of incapacitating symptoms or asymptomatic arrhythmias.

ECG data preceding and following an event are transmitted to monitoring centers by telephone, WiFi, or Bluetooth connection. ELRs may be triggered manually by patients on symptom onset or automatically by device algorithms, enabling the capture of both symptomatic and asymptomatic arrhythmias.[22] Patient tolerance of ELRs may be limited by continuous use of electrodes during the monitoring period, whereas transmission of recordings may be difficult for patients who are unfamiliar with technology or live alone.[23]

ELRs have high utility in the investigation of clinical symptoms suspicious for arrhythmia. The SYNARR-Flash study found 4-week ELR monitoring to have high diagnostic yield for syncope (24.5%) and palpitations (71.6%), supporting the use of ELRs as a first-line AECG modality in the investigation of syncope or palpitations.[24] In another randomized study of patients presenting with syncope or presyncope, a diagnosis or exclusion of arrhythmia was made in 63% of patients with ELRs compared with 24% of patients with Holter devices ($P<.0001$).[25] Symptom-rhythm correlation in the same study was 56% with ELRs compared with 22% with Holter monitors ($P<.0001$). Indications for ELR use are summarized in **Table 2**.

Mobile Cardiac Telemetry

MCT devices are the newest-generation AECG modality, offering the advantages of both continuous and event-based recording and allowing real-time data monitoring by clinicians using WiFi or cellular networking.[1] Event capture is secondary to both manual triggering and automated rhythm analysis algorithms. MCT devices can therefore generate patient and caregiver alarms in real time in response to detected arrhythmias.[26] Depending on the device, single-lead or 3-lead monitoring may be possible. Because of their novelty, MCT devices are generally more expensive and less widely available than Holter monitors, event recorders, or ELRs.[27]

MCT has been associated with an increased diagnostic yield compared with other modalities of AECG monitoring. In a 2007 randomized control trial, Rothman and colleagues[22] found that diagnosis of arrhythmia following unsuccessful 24-hour Holter monitoring was made in 88% of MCT-monitored patients, compared with 75% of patients monitored with loop event monitors ($P = .008$). A 2013 retrospective analysis comparing MCT with Holter and event monitoring showed a higher diagnostic yield with MCT (61%) than event (23%) or Holter monitoring (24%).[26] In addition, more patients monitored by MCT are initiated on antiarrhythmic drugs. A

2013 retrospective analysis indicated initiation of therapy in 61% of patients diagnosed by MCT compared with 39% of event and 43% of Holter-monitored patients.[26] Indications for MCT use are summarized in **Table 2**.

DISCUSSION
General Principles in Device Selection

Device selection for AECG monitoring should encompass patient, clinician, and health care system considerations.[1] Appropriate selection should involve clinical factors, including modality-specific diagnostic sensitivity and specificity, expected or hypothesized frequency of arrhythmic events, and estimated risk to patients of adverse events secondary to arrhythmia. Patient-specific factors, including access to health care, adherence to AECG recording, and expected cost, should ideally be considered in order to increase diagnostic yield and effectiveness. In addition, the ability of individual health care systems to provide and collect AECG devices and interpret their recordings varies widely, often limiting the selection of various devices.

Indications for Ambulatory External Electrocardiography Monitoring

Clinical indications
Palpitations AECG monitoring is indicated where initial clinical investigations (history, physical examination, standard 12-lead ECG) fail to identify a cause of the palpitations, or if they suggest arrhythmia as an underlying cause.[24] Holter monitors used for 24-hour and 48-hour periods have low diagnostic yield and symptom-rhythm correlation in patients presenting with palpitations, although they may be appropriate in patients with frequent or reproducible symptoms or in patients older than 50 years.[28,29] In patients who have less frequent symptoms, extended Holter monitoring may be considered, although there is little evidence supporting increased diagnostic yield compared with 24-hour or 48-hour monitoring in the assessment of palpitations. In light of evidence supporting their preferential use rather than Holter monitors, ELRs or MCT should be considered as first-line investigations where appropriate.[24,27]

Syncope Multiple evidence-based risk scores are useful in estimating the short-term morbidity and mortality in patients presenting with syncope; clinical assessment suggesting a high risk should warrant inpatient admission for further investigations.[30,31] Low-risk patients may be adequately managed with outpatient investigations for a cause of their syncope, including AECG.[32,33] As with the investigation of palpitations, diagnostic yield in syncope is proportional to monitoring duration.[34] ELRs (with automated triggering capability) and MCT monitoring offer higher diagnostic yield than Holter monitors in this setting.[27,34]

The use of patient-triggered devices (event recorders, certain ELRs) that do not offer continuous recording or automatically record arrhythmic episodes is extremely limited in patients presenting with nonprodromal syncope, because sudden incapacitation prevents their activation.

Chest pain The role of AECG in the investigation of chest pain (for a new diagnosis of coronary artery disease [CAD]) is likely limited. Transient, asymptomatic episodes of ST-segment deviation may be identified by nonstress AECG, but the clinical value of capturing these episodes is unclear. Nair and colleagues[35] found the specificity of ST-segment deviation on ambulatory Holter monitoring predicting CAD to be 91%, although it was poorly sensitive (19%), suggesting a limited use for AECG in the clinical exclusion of ischemic cardiac disease. ST-segment deviation in the same study was not a predictor of all-cause mortality or future cardiac events.

In patients with known (angiographically diagnosed) CAD, AECG monitoring may have greater clinical utility. Silent ischemia, or transient ST-segment depression (captured on AECG) without anginal symptoms, has been clinically recognized in patients with stable and unstable CAD as a marker of poor prognosis.[36] A lack of large-scale studies examining the utility of eliminating or reducing silent ischemia as a treatment goal has prevented the more widespread use of AECG for this purpose, although this may change as devices become more inexpensive and frequently used.

Analysis of ST-segment depression on AECG may be used to stratify future cardiac risk following acute myocardial infarction, although this is not routine practice. In patients with ST-elevation myocardial infarction following primary PCI, ST-segment recovery assessed by Holter monitoring predicts both overall mortality and the infarct size assessed by sestamibi imaging.[37] Analysis of AECGs from patients enrolled in the DANAMI-2 trial found that the presence of ST-segment elevation on AECG predicted mortality and major cardiac events in patients who were treated with fibrinolysis following ST-elevation myocardial infarction.[38]

Diagnosis of atrial fibrillation

AF is associated with significant morbidity and mortality; increasing risk of heart failure, dementia, and 4-fold to 5-fold increased risk of stroke have been independently associated with AF in multiple studies.[39] Timely diagnosis allows early initiation of risk-reducing therapy, and the utility of AECG for this purpose is well documented in multiple clinical settings.[17]

Atrial fibrillation in patients with cryptogenic stroke Perhaps one of the most well-studied uses of AECG for the diagnosis of AF is in patients following stroke of unknown cause (cryptogenic stroke). Although there is no evidence supporting indefinite oral anticoagulation (OAC) in this population, subsequent diagnosis of AF suggests an embolic mechanism of stroke and therefore identifies an indication for OAC. AECG is widely used as part of standard investigation in all patients with cryptogenic stroke, with Holter monitors being the most commonly used.[40]

The diagnostic yield obtained with external AECG in current literature varies widely. This variation is partly caused by a lack of consensus regarding the minimum AF duration required for diagnosis and treatment. In the EMBRACE randomized controlled trial assessing AF diagnostic yield in 30-day event monitoring versus 24-hour Holter monitoring, paroxysmal AF was common (12.3% of all patients), especially in patients aged 55 years or older.[41] Changing the definition from greater than or equal to 2.5 minutes to greater than or equal to 30 seconds resulted in an increase in diagnostic yield from 2.5% to 3.2% and 9.9% to 16.1% in Holter and event monitor groups, respectively.

Regardless of minimum AF duration, evidence supports increased diagnostic yield in these patients with increasing duration of monitoring. To this end, the highest diagnostic yield is generally observed with insertable cardiac monitors. The CRYSTAL-AF trial randomized patients with cryptogenic stroke and 24 hours of unsuccessful ECG monitoring to insertable cardiac monitoring or standard follow-up based on local practice.[42] Results indicated superiority of insertable cardiac monitors to conventional follow-up, with diagnostic yields of 12.4% and 2% at 12 months, respectively. Evidence from similar studies suggests an increased diagnostic yield associated with monitoring beyond 24 hours and until 30 days, although data suggesting a superiority of early initiation of long-term (ie, >30 days) monitoring to 30 day monitoring are lacking.[8,40]

Procedures or lengthy follow-up required by insertable monitors are not accepted by some patients, who prefer external devices instead. A 2016 analysis of existing literature found diagnostic yield obtained with Holter monitoring to range between 1.7% and 27.3%; 3 of 16 studies monitored patients for more than 3 days.[8] Yield was higher with ELRs and MCT, although duration of monitoring with either was rarely less than 21 days. Beyond extension of monitoring duration, the most compelling argument for the use of any specific AECG modality is estimated patient adherence. Decisions on AECG monitoring in this setting must take clinical factors, device availability, cost, and patient behaviors into account.

Evidence exists to support a stepwise approach to monitoring. Sposato and colleagues[43] conducted a systematic review and meta-analysis evaluating diagnostic yield of novel AF in patients following stroke with 4 phases of monitoring: emergency department 12-lead ECG; serial 12-lead ECG, Holter, or cardiac telemetry during admission; outpatient ambulatory Holter; and outpatient MCT, event monitoring, or implantable monitoring. This method resulted in an overall yield of 23.7% following all phases of monitoring and provides a cost-effective framework for the use of AECG in this setting.

Use in proarrhythmic syndromes

Long QT syndrome Long QT syndrome (LQTS) represents a group of genetic channelopathies that cause prolongation of the QT interval associated with an increased risk of arrhythmia and cardiac arrest. AECG has long held a role in diagnostic confirmation of LQTS and may have a role in risk stratification as well.

The capture of ECG data from multiple emotional, activity, and autonomic states may allow some risk stratification for patients with LQTS. Among patients with LQTS, prolonged corrected QT and adaption of QT to changes in heart rate predict risk of future cardiac events in patients with LQT1 and LQT2 mutations.[44–46] In a small group of patients, vagal and sympathetic control (based on analysis of diurnal R-R and QT interval variation) were found to correlate with future arrhythmic risk in patients carrying 1 LQT1 mutation.[47]

Monitoring following antiarrhythmic intervention

Pharmacotherapy Quantitative reduction in the number of PVCs and frequency of nonsustained ventricular tachycardia (NSVT) have long been measured as markers of ventricular antiarrhythmic drug efficacy. Early consensus on the use of Holter monitors in this setting suggested a reduction of PVCs by 75% and NSVT by 90% to indicate successful arrhythmic suppression.[48] AECG has not commonly been used to measure the efficacy of antiarrhythmic drugs in the suppression of atrial arrhythmias.

AECG may also be used for the monitoring of adverse effects related to antiarrhythmic drug administration, including QT prolongation, spontaneous arrhythmia, and symptomatic or asymptomatic bradycardia. There is a lack of evidence supporting preferential use of any specific AECG device for monitoring in such patients. Diagnostic yield of both adverse effects and persistent arrhythmia may increase with prolonged monitoring, but there is no consensus on a minimum accepted monitoring duration. The pursuit of extended monitoring should therefore be guided by clinical judgment along with local practice standards.

Ablative therapy Monitoring following catheter or surgical ablation is simply and effectively achieved with AECG. In patients receiving ablation for ventricular arrhythmia, surveillance for recurrence with either 24-hour to 72-hour Holter or 30-day event monitoring every 6 months for at least 6 to 12 months is recommended by consensus statements.[49] The use of antiarrhythmic drugs following ablation is unstandardized, but outpatient AECG may have additional utility for monitoring in patients who continue them postprocedure.

Ablation is also a widely used intervention for treatment-refractory AF. Recurrence of AF or atrial tachycardia (AT) is difficult to predict and is common in the early so-called blanking period, although this is difficult to correlate to long-term recurrence and is not always an indication for treatment. AECG monitoring is well studied in long-term follow-up after AF ablation. Evidence from multiple studies suggests AECG monitoring 6 months postablation for extended durations (7–30 days) is significantly superior to monitoring for less than 5 days.[50] In patients with no detected recurrence by AECG, cessation of OAC can be considered, although expert opinion suggests embolic risk may persist even in sinus rhythm if atrial contraction is impaired on functional imaging.[51]

Device therapy Modern pacemakers and implantable cardiac defibrillators (ICDs) have lifetime memory as well as event monitoring–like functionality, reducing the need for additional AECG studies. Captured ECGs from intracardiac leads are generally limited to vectors approximating limb leads (I, II, and III on 12-lead setups), depending on the exact number and location of pacing or ICD leads.[52] This limitation prevents the interpretation of positional or morphologic diagnoses such as the localization of ischemia or hypertrophy. Furthermore, the lack of recording capability while pacing means that pacemaker/ICD recordings do not show loss of capture.

Use of AECG in patients with implanted pacemaker or ICDs is therefore limited mainly to investigation of symptoms suggestive of physical device malfunction (eg, loss of capture, lead malposition) or previously undiagnosed arrhythmia. AECG can verify (1) appropriate pacemaker inhibition; (2) myocardial capture during active pacing; (3) depolarization of the appropriate electrical structures; and (4) appropriate activation of device functions, such as overdrive pacing or ICD shock.

The diagnosis of novel arrhythmia in patients with pacemakers or ICDs has significant clinical impact. For example, a diagnosis of AF in a patient with cardiac resynchronization therapy can explain clinical deterioration despite appropriate device function; such a clinical course should prompt surface ECG investigation if not AECG. New AF also allows risk reduction with OAC as in other patients without implanted devices. Internal device capture is very sensitive for the detection of AF. Israel and colleagues[53] found diagnostic yield with pacemakers and ICDs to be 88% compared with 46% with surface ECGs among patients with a documented history of AF on antiarrhythmic drug therapy. Nonetheless, superior positional inference allowed by surface ECG leads may allow more detailed characterization of atrial arrhythmias, especially in complex cases.

Other indications

Holter-based monitoring parameters The large amount of data obtained by Holter monitors allows the calculation of multiple markers useful for risk stratification, autonomic nervous tone, or diagnosis of arrhythmia. These parameters are only obtained with the use of continuous monitors and dedicated analysis software but may offer some clinical value in patients poorly captured by guideline or consensus statements.

HRT describes the cyclic variation of heart rate following a PVC. Physiologically, abnormal HRT serves as an indirect measure of baroreceptor sensitivity and has been correlated with increased risk in multiple independent studies, although it has not been widely adopted into clinical practice. HRT has utility for risk stratification in patients after myocardial infarction, where both abnormal HRT and turbulence slope (TS) values are associated with arrhythmia and sudden cardiac death.[54,55] In patients with heart failure, particularly with moderately reduced left ventricular ejection fraction, abnormal HRT and TS have been associated with increased sudden cardiac death, all-cause mortality, and progression of heart failure.[56]

HRV describes the amount of variation in R-R intervals observed with continuous ECG monitoring.[57] The amount of HRV, often described as the standard deviation of N-N intervals (SDNN), reflects whole-body autonomic regulation of sympathetic and parasympathetic systems. Depressed HRV has been correlated with increased mortality in multiple systemic disorders, including sepsis, hemodialysis, and liver cirrhosis.[58–60] In patients following myocardial infarction, depressed HRV is a predictor of mortality and arrhythmic events.[54,55] In patients with heart failure, reduction in SDNN is a powerful predictor of mortality caused by heart failure progression.[61]

Novel and Emerging Indications

Cardiac monitoring in the time of coronavirus disease 2019

The emergence of coronavirus disease 2019 (COVID-19) in early 2020 had profound effects on health care systems worldwide, causing both increased admissions to hospital for critical care and decreased presentations to care by patients concerned for an increased risk of infectious exposure.

Early analyses indicated a large burden of arrhythmia observed in patients admitted to hospital for COVID-19 in Wuhan, China.[62] Cardiac injury (denoted by cardiac troponin I [cTnI] levels greater than the upper limit of normal) was also observed in 14.7% of patients with cTnI measured on admission. Within this group, 25.9% had documented arrhythmia. The association of arrhythmia and COVID-19 has been continually reportedly in small observational reports, but the true burden of arrhythmia is unknown, especially in the outpatient setting. Suggested mechanisms of arrhythmia include myocarditis, systemic inflammation, increased cardiac demand caused by systemic illness, and effects of pharmacotherapy used in the management of COVID-19.[63] At this time, the utility of AECG monitoring in patients with COVID-19 is unclear.

The utility of AECG in allowing outpatient investigation and management of arrhythmia is further increased in the current setting of the COVID-19 pandemic. All AECG modalities may be used without significant patient exposure to health care settings, either through postage return of devices to assessment centers or by upload of data to remote monitoring centers. Follow-up with patients can be conducted virtually by telehealth appointment, and infectious risk can therefore be minimized.

SUMMARY

The development of external AECG technology has resulted in a wide variety of available devices and modalities. Few recommendations or guidelines exist favoring one modality more than another, although evidence suggests newer-generation modalities (ELRs, MCT) have superior diagnostic yield in most settings compared with other external AECG modalities (Holter, event recorders). Some evidence exists for a stepwise approach to monitoring to maximize diagnostic yield and minimize cost, but only in the context of monitoring following cryptogenic stroke. For other indications, clinicians should use AECG with patient and clinical factors in mind. Future developments may allow more widespread availability of MCT technology and result in a new standard of care in external AECG monitoring.

CLINICS CARE POINTS

- Extended cardiac monitoring is essential for symptom-rhythm correlation.
- Extended cardiac monitoring allows qualitative and quantitative analysis of cardiac arrhythmias.

DISCLOSURE

The authors have nothing to disclose.

REFERENCES

1. Steinberg JS, Varma N, Cygankiewicz I, et al. 2017 ISHNE-HRS expert consensus statement on ambulatory ECG and external cardiac monitoring/telemetry. Ann Noninvasive Electrocardiol 2017;22(3): e12447.
2. Mond HG. The spectrum of ambulatory electrocardiographic monitoring. Heart Lung Circ 2017; 26(11):1160–74.
3. Holter NJ, Generelli JA. Remote recording of physiological data by radio. Rocky Mt Med J 1949;46(9): 747–51.
4. Kennedy HL. The evolution of ambulatory ECG monitoring. Prog Cardiovasc Dis 2013;56(2):127–32.
5. Enriquez A, Bittner A, Almehairi M, et al. Electrophysiology study without intracardiac catheters. The value of proper Holter interpretation: a case report. J Electrocardiol 2014;47(3):329–32.
6. Longo D, Baranchuk A. Premature ventricular contraction-induced concealed retrograde penetration: electrocardiographic manifestations on anterograde ventricular preexcitation. Ann Noninvasive Electrocardiol 2018;23(2):e12488.
7. Diez JCL, Michael KA, Rocchinotti M, et al. Concealed antegrade penetration of the atrioventricular node. Int J Cardiol 2011;149(3):e125–6.
8. De Angelis G, Cimon K, Sinclair A, et al. Monitoring for atrial fibrillation in discharged stroke and transient ischemic attack patients: a clinical and cost-effectiveness analysis and review of patient preferences. CADTH Optim Use Rep 2016;148.
9. Schuchert A, Behrens G, Meinertz T. Impact of long-term ECG recording on the detection of paroxysmal atrial fibrillation in patients after an acute ischemic stroke. Pacing Clin Electrophysiol PACE 1999; 22(7):1082–4.
10. Barrett PM, Komatireddy R, Haaser S, et al. Comparison of 24-hour Holter monitoring with 14-day novel adhesive patch electrocardiographic monitoring. Am J Med 2014;127(1):95.e11–7.
11. Chua S-K, Chen L-C, Lien L-M, et al. Comparison of arrhythmia detection by 24-hour holter and 14-day continuous electrocardiography patch monitoring. Acta Cardiol Sin 2020;36(3):251–9.
12. Lobodzinski SS. ECG patch monitors for assessment of cardiac rhythm abnormalities. Prog Cardiovasc Dis 2013;56(2):224–9.
13. Loring Z, Hanna P, Pellegrini CN. Longer ambulatory ECG monitoring increases identification of clinically significant ectopy. Pacing Clin Electrophysiol PACE 2016;39(6):592–7.
14. Mittal S. The evaluation of the patient with unexplained palpitations: maximizing diagnostic yield while minimizing unnecessary frustration. Ann Noninvasive Electrocardiol 2015;20(6):515–7.
15. Dussault C, Toeg H, Nathan M, et al. Electrocardiographic monitoring for detecting atrial fibrillation after ischemic stroke or transient ischemic attack: systematic review and meta-analysis. Circ Arrhythm Electrophysiol 2015;8(2):263–9.
16. Tung CE, Su D, Turakhia MP, et al. Diagnostic yield of extended cardiac patch monitoring in patients with stroke or TIA. Front Neurol 2014;5:266.
17. Hariri E, Hachem A, Sarkis G, et al. Optimal duration of monitoring for atrial fibrillation in cryptogenic stroke: a nonsystematic review. Biomed Res Int 2016;2016:5704963.
18. Fogel RI, Evans JJ, Prystowsky EN. Utility and cost of event recorders in the diagnosis of palpitations, presyncope, and syncope. Am J Cardiol 1997; 79(2):207–8.
19. Wu C-C, Hsieh M-H, Tai C-T, et al. Utility of patient-activated cardiac event recorders in the detection of cardiac arrhythmias. J Interv Card Electrophysiol Int J Arrhythm Pacing 2003;8(2):117–20.
20. Scalvini S, Zanelli E, Martinelli G, et al. Cardiac event recording yields more diagnoses than 24-hour Holter monitoring in patients with palpitations. J Telemed Telecare 2005;11(Suppl 1):14–6.
21. Kohno R, Abe H, Benditt DG. Ambulatory electrocardiogram monitoring devices for evaluating transient loss of consciousness or other related symptoms. J Arrhythmia 2017;33(6):583–9.

22. Rothman SA, Laughlin JC, Seltzer J, et al. The diagnosis of cardiac arrhythmias: a prospective multicenter randomized study comparing mobile cardiac outpatient telemetry versus standard loop event monitoring. J Cardiovasc Electrophysiol 2007;18(3):241–7.

23. Gula LJ, Krahn AD, Massel D, et al. External loop recorders: determinants of diagnostic yield in patients with syncope. Am Heart J 2004;147(4):644–8.

24. Locati ET, Moya A, Oliveira M, et al. External prolonged electrocardiogram monitoring in unexplained syncope and palpitations: results of the SYNARR-Flash study. Europace 2016;18(8):1265–72.

25. Sivakumaran S, Krahn AD, Klein GJ, et al. A prospective randomized comparison of loop recorders versus Holter monitors in patients with syncope or presyncope. Am J Med 2003;115(1):1–5.

26. Tsang J-P, Mohan S. Benefits of monitoring patients with mobile cardiac telemetry (MCT) compared with the Event or Holter monitors. Med Devices Auckl NZ 2013;7:1–5.

27. Olson JA, Fouts AM, Padanilam BJ, et al. Utility of mobile cardiac outpatient telemetry for the diagnosis of palpitations, presyncope, syncope, and the assessment of therapy efficacy. J Cardiovasc Electrophysiol 2007;18(5):473–7.

28. Irfan G, Ahmad M, Khan AR. Association between symptoms and frequency of arrhythmias on 24-hour Holter monitoring. J Coll Physicians Surg Pak 2009;19(11):686–9.

29. Paudel B, Paudel K. The diagnostic significance of the holter monitoring in the evaluation of palpitation. J Clin Diagn Res 2013;7(3):480–3.

30. Reed MJ. Approach to syncope in the emergency department. Emerg Med J 2019;36(2):108–16.

31. Barón-Esquivias G, Fernández-Cisnal A, Arce-León Á, et al. Prognosis of patients with syncope seen in the emergency room department: an evaluation of four different risk scores recommended by the European Society of Cardiology guidelines. Eur J Emerg Med 2017;24(6):428–34.

32. Runser LA, Gauer RL, Houser A. Syncope: evaluation and differential diagnosis. Am Fam Physician 2017;95(5):303–12.

33. Puppala VK, Dickinson O, Benditt DG. Syncope: classification and risk stratification. J Cardiol 2014;63(3):171–7.

34. Cheung CC, Krahn AD. Loop recorders for syncope evaluation: what is the evidence? Expert Rev Med Devices 2016;13(11):1021–7.

35. Nair CK, Khan IA, Esterbrooks DJ, et al. Diagnostic and prognostic value of Holter-detected ST-segment deviation in unselected patients with chest pain referred for coronary angiography: a long-term follow-up analysis. Chest 2001;120(3):834–9.

36. Wimmer NJ, Scirica BM, Stone PH. The clinical significance of continuous ECG (ambulatory ECG or Holter) monitoring of the ST-segment to evaluate ischemia: a review. Prog Cardiovasc Dis 2013;56(2):195–202.

37. Kuijt WJ, Green CL, Verouden NJW, et al. What is the best ST-segment recovery parameter to predict clinical outcome and myocardial infarct size? Amplitude, speed, and completeness of ST-segment recovery after primary percutaneous coronary intervention for ST-segment elevation myocardial infarction. J Electrocardiol 2017;50(6):952–9.

38. Idorn L, Høfsten DE, Wachtell K, et al, DANAMI-2 Investigators. Prevalence and prognostic implications of ST-segment deviations from ambulatory Holter monitoring after ST-segment elevation myocardial infarction treated with either fibrinolysis or primary percutaneous coronary intervention (a Danish Trial in Acute Myocardial Infarction-2 Substudy). Am J Cardiol 2007;100(6):937–43.

39. Kornej J, Börschel CS, Benjamin EJ, et al. Epidemiology of atrial fibrillation in the 21st century: novel methods and new insights. Circ Res 2020;127(1):4–20.

40. Albers GW, Bernstein RA, Brachmann J, et al. Heart rhythm monitoring strategies for cryptogenic stroke: 2015 diagnostics and monitoring stroke focus group report. J Am Heart Assoc 2016;5(3):e002944.

41. Gladstone DJ, Spring M, Dorian P, et al. Atrial fibrillation in patients with cryptogenic stroke. N Engl J Med 2014;370(26):2467–77.

42. Sanna T, Diener H-C, Passman RS, et al. Cryptogenic stroke and underlying atrial fibrillation. N Engl J Med 2014;370(26):2478–86.

43. Sposato LA, Cipriano LE, Saposnik G, et al. Diagnosis of atrial fibrillation after stroke and transient ischaemic attack: a systematic review and meta-analysis. Lancet Neurol 2015;14(4):377–87.

44. Priori SG, Schwartz PJ, Napolitano C, et al. Risk stratification in the long-QT syndrome. N Engl J Med 2003;348(19):1866–74.

45. Mathias A, Moss AJ, Lopes CM, et al. Prognostic implications of mutation-specific QTc standard deviation in congenital long QT syndrome. Heart Rhythm 2013;10(5):720–5.

46. Page A, McNitt S, Xia X, et al. Population-based beat-to-beat QT analysis from Holter recordings in the long QT syndrome. J Electrocardiol 2017;50(6):787–91.

47. Porta A, Girardengo G, Bari V, et al. Autonomic control of heart rate and QT interval variability influences arrhythmic risk in long QT syndrome type 1. J Am Coll Cardiol 2015;65(4):367–74.

48. Morganroth J. Evaluation of antiarrhythmic therapy using Holter monitoring. Am J Cardiol 1988;62(12):18H–23H.

49. Cronin EM, Bogun FM, Maury P, et al. 2019 HRS/EHRA/APHRS/LAHRS expert consensus statement on catheter ablation of ventricular arrhythmias. Europace 2019;21(8):1143–4.

50. Ajijola OA, Boyle NG, Shivkumar K. Detecting and monitoring arrhythmia recurrence following catheter

ablation of atrial fibrillation. Front Physiol 2015;6. https://doi.org/10.3389/fphys.2015.00090.

51. Anselmino M, Rovera C, Marchetto G, et al. Antico-agulant cessation following atrial fibrillation ablation: limits of the ECG-guided approach. Expert Rev Cardiovasc Ther 2017;15(6):473–9.

52. Diemberger I, Gardini B, Martignani C, et al. Holter ECG for pacemaker/defibrillator carriers: what is its role in the era of remote monitoring? Heart Br Card Soc 2015;101(16):1272–8.

53. Israel CW, Grönefeld G, Ehrlich JR, et al. Long-term risk of recurrent atrial fibrillation as documented by an implantable monitoring device: implications for optimal patient care. J Am Coll Cardiol 2004;43(1):47–52.

54. Exner DV, Kavanagh KM, Slawnych MP, et al. Noninvasive risk assessment early after a myocardial infarction the REFINE study. J Am Coll Cardiol 2007;50(24):2275–84.

55. Huikuri HV, Exner DV, Kavanagh KM, et al. Attenuated recovery of heart rate turbulence early after myocardial infarction identifies patients at high risk for fatal or near-fatal arrhythmic events. Heart Rhythm 2010;7(2):229–35.

56. Cygankiewicz I. Heart rate turbulence. Prog Cardiovasc Dis 2013;56(2):160–71.

57. Electrophysiology Task Force of the European Society of Cardiology, The North American Society of Pacing. Heart rate variability. Circulation 1996; 93(5):1043–65.

58. de Castilho FM, Ribeiro ALP, Nobre V, et al. Heart rate variability as predictor of mortality in sepsis: a systematic review. PLoS One 2018;13(9):e0203487.

59. Kuo G, Chen S-W, Huang J-Y, et al. Short-term heart rate variability as a predictor of long-term survival in patients with chronic hemodialysis: a prospective cohort study. J Formos Med Assoc Taiwan Yi Zhi 2018;117(12):1058–64.

60. Bhogal AS, De Rui M, Pavanello D, et al. Which heart rate variability index is an independent predictor of mortality in cirrhosis? Dig Liver Dis 2019;51(5): 695–702.

61. Nolan J, Batin PD, Andrews R, et al. Prospective study of heart rate variability and mortality in chronic heart failure: results of the United Kingdom heart failure evaluation and assessment of risk trial (UK-heart). Circulation 1998;98(15):1510–6.

62. Si D, Du B, Ni L, et al. Death, discharge and arrhythmias among patients with COVID-19 and cardiac injury. CMAJ 2020;192(28):E791–8.

63. Dherange P, Lang J, Qian P, et al. Arrhythmias and COVID-19. Jacc Clin Electrophysiol 2020;6(9): 1193–204.

Implantable Loop Recorders—Syncope, Cryptogenic Stroke, Atrial Fibrillation

Suneet Mittal, MD, FACC, FHRS[a,b,*]

KEYWORDS

- Arrhythmia • Atrial fibrillation • Cryptogenic stroke • Implantable loop recorder
- Insertable cardiac monitor • Monitoring • Syncope

KEY POINTS

- Current guidelines have identified distinct populations with unexplained syncope who may benefit from an implantable loop recorder for long-term electrocardiographic monitoring.
- In patients with cryptogenic stroke, empirical anticoagulation has not been shown to be helpful. Thus, implantable loop recorders have been recommended to identify patients who have atrial fibrillation.
- Patients with cryptogenic stroke in whom an implantable loop recorder detects atrial fibrillation may benefit from initiation of anticoagulation; however, the threshold for atrial fibrillation duration that should trigger this is currently unknown.
- In patients with known atrial fibrillation, implantable loop recorders allow for the precise determination of pattern, number, duration, and burden of these episodes as well as the ventricular rate during atrial fibrillation.
- Current devices have certain software and hardware limitations that need to be improved to facilitate optimal utility of these devices.

The implantable loop recorder (ILR) is a subcutaneous, single-lead, electrocardiographic (ECG) monitoring device used for diagnosis in patients with recurrent, unexplained episodes of palpitations or syncope, for long-term monitoring in patients at risk for atrial fibrillation (AF), and to guide clinical management in patients with known AF.[1] These devices are capable of storing and transmitting ECG data automatically in response to a significant bradyarrhythmia or tachyarrhythmia or in response to patient activation, and this makes them particularly useful either when symptoms are infrequent or when aggregate long-term ECG data are necessary. The aim of this document is to review the clinical utility of

ILRs for arrhythmia monitoring in common clinical situations.

SYNCOPE

Syncope is defined as a transient loss of consciousness due to global cerebral hypoperfusion and is characterized by rapid onset, short duration, and spontaneous complete recovery. It is an extremely common clinical problem and often has an underlying cardiovascular cause. The initial evaluation of syncope consists of a comprehensive history, physical examination (including orthostatic blood pressure measurements), and an ECG. This initial evaluation dictates the decision

[a] Department of Cardiology, Snyder Center for Comprehensive Atrial Fibrillation, Valley Health System, Ridgewood, NJ, USA; [b] Electrophysiology, Valley Health System, 970 Linwood Avenue, Paramus, NJ 07652, USA
* Electrophysiology, Valley Health System, 970 Linwood Avenue, Paramus, NJ 07652.
E-mail address: mittsu@valleyhealth.com

Card Electrophysiol Clin 13 (2021) 439–447
https://doi.org/10.1016/j.ccep.2021.04.006

on whether hospitalization is necessary for further evaluation as well as the need for additional diagnostic testing.

Because recurrent syncope occurs sporadically and because ECG documentation at the time of recurrent syncope is an extremely important diagnostic modality, ILRs have a significantly greater diagnostic yield than 24-hour Holter, 30-day event, or 30-day mobile cardiovascular telemetry monitoring.[2] The diagnostic yield of any ECG monitoring strategy increases as the monitoring period is increased; ILRs (with their several year battery life) offer the best opportunity for diagnosis. The PICTURE registry was a prospective, multicenter, observational study that followed-up 570 patients with recurrent unexplained pre-syncope or syncope who received an ILR. It was shown that these patients were evaluated on average by 3 different specialists and underwent a median of 13 nondiagnostic tests (range 9–20). Within the first year, syncope recurred in one-third of the patients; the ILR provided a diagnosis in 78% of the patients, most commonly a cardiac cause.[3]

Current American College of Cardiology/American Heart Association/Heart Rhythm Society guidelines for the evaluation and management of patients with syncope acknowledge, "the choice of monitoring system and duration should be appropriate to the likelihood that a spontaneous event will be detected and the patient may be incapacitated and unable to voluntarily trigger the recording system".[4] These guidelines also recommend "to evaluate selected ambulatory patients with syncope of suspected arrhythmic etiology, an insertable cardiac monitor can be useful"; the recommendation carries a IIa class of recommendation and B-R level (quality) of evidence (**Fig. 1**). The European Society of Cardiology guidelines on the other hand are more supportive of the use of ILRs in patients with unexplained syncope. In fact, they identify 2 separate class I

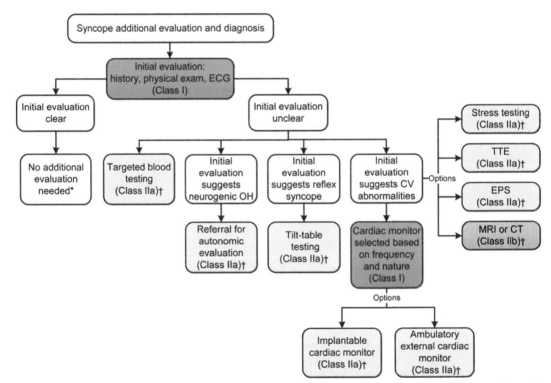

Fig. 1. Evaluation and diagnosis for syncope. *Applies to patients after a normal initial evaluation without significant injury or cardiovascular morbidities; patients followed-up by primary care physician as needed. †In selected patients. CT computed tomography; CV, cardiovascular; ECG, electrocardiogram; EPS, electrophysiological study; OH, orthostatic hypotension; and TTE, transthoracic echocardiography. (*From* Shen W-K, Sheldon RS, Benditt DG, Cohen MI, Forman DE, Goldberger ZD, Grubb BP, Hamdan MH, Krahn AD, Link MS, Olshansky B, Raj SR, Sandhu RK, Sorajja D, Sun BC, Yancy CW. 2017 ACC/AHA/HRS guideline for the evaluation and management of patients with syncope: a report of the American College of Cardiology/American Heart Association Task Force on Clinical Practice Guidelines and the Heart Rhythm Society. *Circulation* 2017; 136: e60–e122. 10.1161/CIR. 0000000000000499; with permission.)

recommendations and 1 class IIa recommendation for use of implantable monitors (**Table 1**).[4-6] The recommendations have been informed by a series of studies performed in various populations with unexplained syncope evaluated using an ILR (**Table 2**).[7-11]

CRYPTOGENIC STROKE

A stroke occurs in approximately 800,000 patients each in the United States alone; despite extensive evaluation, a definitive cause cannot be identified in 10% to 40% of patients. These patients are considered to have had a cryptogenic stroke. AF is a common cause for stroke; because anticoagulation is effective in reducing the risk of stroke in patients with AF, it was natural to consider anticoagulation in patients with cryptogenic stroke. However, 2 randomized clinical trials have failed to show the clinical benefit of such a strategy.[12,13]

Therefore, ECG monitoring to detect AF has been recommended in patients with cryptogenic stroke. The 2020 European Society of Cardiology guidelines on the management of AF advocate short- and long-term ECG monitoring in these

patients (**Table 3**).[14] In the authors' experience, these patients all undergo an ECG on presentation and then are maintained on hospital telemetry while undergoing a standard evaluation to determine a cause for stroke and define a strategy for treatment.

In randomized clinical trials, both ambulatory external ECG (AECG) monitoring and ILRs have been shown to subsequently increase the likelihood of detecting AF as compared with usual follow-up.[15,16] The unresolved question is whether AECG monitoring should be performed first in all patients with cryptogenic stroke, followed, if needed, by an ILR, or whether an ILR should be implanted before hospital discharge in these patients in lieu of any additional AECG monitoring. Each approach has its inherent benefits and limitations (**Table 4**); the reality is the likelihood of detecting AF in the first 30 days following a cryptogenic stroke is only about 5%. Furthermore, episodes are typically paroxysmal and constitute a very low (<1%) overall burden of AF.[17]

CRYSTAL-AF was a randomized clinical trial that compared an ILR (n = 221) with conventional follow-up (n = 220) in patients with cryptogenic stroke.[16] Patients were older than 40 years and had a cryptogenic stroke within the previous 90 days. The primary endpoint of the study was the time to first detection of AF within 6 months; a secondary endpoint was the time to first detection of AF within the first 12 months. At 6 and 12-month post-ILR implant, AF was detected in 8.9% and 12.4% of patients, respectively, who had received an ILR; this was 6.4 and 7.3 times, respectively, more likely than patients managed through conventional follow-up. By 3 years of follow-up, 30% of patients in the ILR had device-detected AF. The median time to an AF episode was 8.4 months; 81% of episodes were asymptomatic and resulted in the initiation of oral anticoagulation in most of the patients.[18] Furthermore, a recent analysis demonstrated that directly proceeding to an ILR in these patients is cost-effective, in comparison to either usual care or starting first with an AECG monitor (**Fig. 2**).[19]

Nonetheless, 2 limitations exist with using an ILR for long-term ECG monitoring in these patients. First, the positive predictive value is low in this population, which generates a high number of false-positive detections.[20] Second, there are no data that define the minimal duration of detected AF that identifies patients who benefit from anticoagulation. This is important because the positive predictive value for AF detection in an ILR improves as duration of AF episode increases. For example, if the detect duration is 2 minutes, the positive predictive value is 26%; in

Table 1 Indications for an implantable loop recorder in patients with unexplained syncope: summary of the European Society of Cardiology guidelines		
ESC Recommendation	**Class**	**Level**
ILR is indicated in an early phase of evaluation in patients with recurrent syncope of uncertain origin, absence of high-risk criteria, and a high likelihood of recurrence within the battery life of the device.	I	A
ILR is indicated in patients with high-risk criteria in whom a comprehensive evaluation did not demonstrate a cause of syncope or lead to a specific treatment and who do not have conventional indications for primary prevention. ICD or pacemaker indication.	I	A
ILR should be considered in patients with suspected or certain reflex syncope presenting with frequent or severe syncopal episodes.	II	B

Abbreviation: ICD, implantable cardioverter defibrillator.

Table 2
The International Study of Syncope of Uncertain Etiology

Trial	Study Population/Design	Patients, n	Key Findings
ISSUE-1	Patients without structural heart disease or with minor cardiac abnormalities that were considered to be without clinical relevance and not suggestive of a cardiac cause of syncope, absence of intraventricular conduction defects, and a negative complete workup including tilt-testing.[7]	82	An ILR-documented syncopal episode occurred in 24 (29%) patients after a median of 105 d (range, 47–226 d). The most frequent finding, which was observed in 11 (46%) of these 24 patients, was ≥1 asystolic pauses (median 31 s; range, 20–44 s).
	Same population as aforementioned but with a positive response to tilt-testing.[7]	29	An ILR-documented syncopal episode occurred in 8 (28%) patients after a median of 59 d (range, 22–98 d). The most frequent finding, which was observed in 5 (62%) of these 8 patients was ≥1 asystolic pauses (median 33 s; range, 23–41 s). No difference in baseline characteristics or follow-up outcomes between patients with and without a positive response to tilt-testing.
	Patients with bundle branch block and a negative electrophysiological test.[8]	52	Syncope recurred in 22 (42%) patients. The most frequent findings, recorded in 17 (77%) patients, was ≥1 prolonged asystolic pause mainly attributable to AV block. AV block not observed in patients with isolated right bundle branch block.
	Patients with overt heart disease who were at risk of ventricular arrhythmia, because these were patients with depressed ejection fraction or nonsustained ventricular tachycardia in whom an electrophysiological study did not induce sustained ventricular arrhythmias.[9]	35	Syncope recurred in 6 (17%) patients after a mean of 6 ± 5 mo. Recurrent syncope was never attributable to a ventricular arrhythmia and never resulted in death.
ISSUE-2	Prospective, multicenter, observational study to assess the efficacy of specific therapy based on ILR diagnostic observations in patients with recurrent suspected neurally medicated syncope.[10]	103	The 1-y recurrence rate in patients assigned to ILR-guided specific therapy was 10%, compared with 41% in the patients without specific therapy. The 1-y recurrence in patients with a pacemaker was 5%.
ISSUE -3	Multicenter, prospective, randomized, double-blind study to evaluate the effectiveness of pacing therapy to prevent recurrent syncope in patients with documented spontaneous asystole during neurally mediated syncope.[11]	77	In patients ≥40 y of age with recurrent asystole (≥3 s + syncope or ≥6 s without syncope) during an episode of neurally mediated syncope, there was a 32% absolute and 57% relative reduction in syncope recurrence. Even with pacing, 25% of patients had recurrent syncope.

Abbreviation: AV, atrioventricular.

Table 3
European Society of Cardiology recommendations for atrial fibrillation monitoring in patients with cryptogenic stroke

ESC Recommendation	Class	Level
In patients with acute ischemic stroke or TIA and without previously known AF, monitoring for AF is recommended using a short-term ECG recording for at least the first 24 h, followed by continuous ECG monitoring for at least 72 h whenever possible.	I	B
In selected stroke patients without previously known AF, additional ECG monitoring using long-term noninvasive ECG monitors or insertable cardiac monitors should be considered, to detect AF.	II	B

Data from Hindricks G, Potpara T, Dagres N, Arbelo E, Bax JJ, Blomström-Lundqvist C, Boriani G, Castella M, Dan G-A, Dilaveris PE, Fauchier L, Filippatos G, Kalman JM, La Meir M, Lane DA, Lebeau J-P, Lettino M, Lip GYH, Pinto FJ, Thomas GN, Valgimigli M, Van Gelder IC, Van Putte BP, Watkins CL, ESC Scientific Document Group, 2020 ESC Guidelines for the diagnosis and management of atrial fibrillation developed in collaboration with the European Association for Cardio-Thoracic Surgery (EACTS): The Task Force for the diagnosis and management of atrial fibrillation of the European Society of Cardiology (ESC) Developed with the special contribution of the European Heart Rhythm Association (EHRA) of the ESC. European Heart Journal, ehaa612, https://doi.org/10.1093/eurheartj/ehaa612.

contrast, if the detect duration is 1 hour, the positive predictive value increases to 91%,[20] which has major implications to workflow and clinical efficiency because a lot of time needs to be spent to adjudicate false-positive episodes.

ATRIAL FIBRILLATION

The utility and limitations of long-term ECG monitoring of AF using an ILR has previously been outlined.[21] ILRs allow for the precise determination of AF pattern, number of AF episodes, the duration and burden of AF episodes, AF density, as well as the ventricular rate during AF (and differentiate this from periods in sinus rhythm). Incorporation of these features into routine clinical practice may positively influence the care of patients with AF.

Accurate characterization of AF allows more homogeneous assignment of patients with AF; this is certainly critical considering patients for clinical therapies and trials. The CIRCA-DOSE study offers important insight into how ILRs can be used in patients with AF. The ultimate aim of this randomized study was to compare the efficacy of cryoballoon and irrigated radiofrequency catheter ablation inpatients with paroxysmal or early persistent AF. All patients were implanted with an ILR at least 30 days before their AF ablation, which allowed the investigators to assess baseline pattern, duration, and burden of AF. Although about half of the patients had a recurrence of AF postablation, the AF burden was reduced by greater than 99%.[22] These data provide strong support of incorporating AF burden as a surrogate of outcome as opposed to a reliance on any recurrence of greater than 30 seconds in duration.

Before ablation, investigators were asked to classify patients based on clinical assessment as having low-burden paroxysmal AF (<4 episodes of AF in past 6 months), high-burden paroxysmal AF (≥4 episodes of AF over the past 6 months with ≥2 episodes >6 hours in duration), or persistent AF. The patients were also classified based on objective data from the ILR. There was poor agreement between clinical and device-based classification of pattern of AF; in addition, clinical assessment did not accurately predict AF burden, postablation AF burden, or freedom from recurrent AF postablation.[23] These data further lend support to the importance of objective assessment of AF pattern before initiating any intervention in order to best understand the impact of any given therapy.

Continuous ECG monitoring also provides an opportunity to consider more granular patterns of AF besides just paroxysmal and persistent. For example, in CIRCA-DOSE, based on ILR data, patients were further stratified into the following groups: the longest AF episode less than 24 hours (n = 263, 76.0%), between 24 and 40 hours (n = 25, 7.2%), between 2 and 7 days (n = 40, 11.7%), and more than 7 days (n = 18, 5.2%). The best outcome following ablation was observed in patients in whom the longest AF episode was less than 24 hours.[24] In addition, the pattern of AF can be quite different between patients. In a recent study where an ILR was implanted in patients undergoing cavotricuspid isthmus ablation for management of typical atrial flutter, 5 distinct patterns of AF were identified (**Fig. 3**)[25]: (1) no AF during follow-up; (2) isolated AF episodes—single AF episode followed by more than 6 months until another AF episode; (3) clusters of AF episodes—more than 1 episode of AF within a month followed by more than 6 months until another AF episode; (4) frequent AF

Table 4
Advantages and disadvantages of two electrocardiographic monitoring strategies in patients with cryptogenic stroke

	Advantages	Disadvantages
Ambulatory external ECG monitoring; if nondiagnostic, move forward with an ILR	• Noninvasive • Can detect AF episodes lasting ≥30 s • Avoid an ILR in patients in whom AF is detected in the first 30 d	• Extended Holter monitors limited to 2 wk of monitoring • MCT monitors can be used for 4 wk but cannot be applied to inpatients in US and not widely available outside the US • If nondiagnostic, there are discontinuities in monitoring while ILR can be implanted
ILR before hospital discharge	• Continuity of monitoring • Provides long-term monitoring • Over time, can ascertain information about AF characteristics (eg, number of episodes, duration, burden, ventricular rates)	• Cannot detect AF <2 min in duration • Low positive predictive value for short episodes in cryptogenic stroke patients • Cost

Abbreviations: MCT, mobile cardiovascular telemetry; US, United States.
Adapted from Milstein NS, Musat DL, Allred J, Seiler A, Pimienta J, Oliveros S, Bhatt AG, Preminger M, Sichrovsky T, Shaw RE, Mittal S. Detection of atrial fibrillation using an implantable loop recorder following cryptogenic stroke: Implications for post-stroke electrocardiographic monitoring. J Interv Card Electrophysiol 2020 Jan; 57(1): 141-147. https://doi.org/10.1007/s10840-019-00628-6. Epub 2019 Oct 14; with permission.

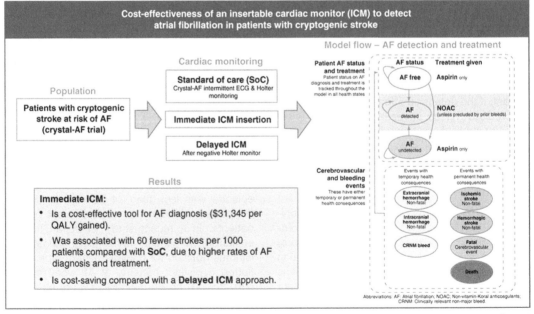

Fig. 2. Cost-effectiveness of an ILR to detect AF in patients with cryptogenic stroke. (*From* Sawyer LM, Witte KK, Reynolds MR, Mittal S, Jones FWG, Rosemas SC, Ziegler PD, Kaplon RE, Yaghi S. Cost–effectiveness of an insertable cardiac monitor to detect atrial fibrillation in patients with cryptogenic stroke. *J Comp Eff Res* 2020 Dec 10. doi: 10.2217/cer-2020-0224; with permission.)

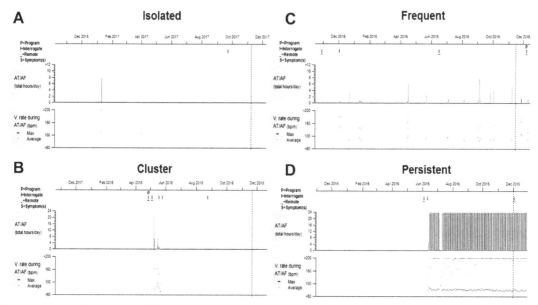

Fig. 3. Patterns of AF and atrial flutter detected by an ILR. (*A*) Isolated: single AF episode followed by more than 6 months until another AF episode. (*B*) Clusters: more than 1 episode of AF within a month followed by more than 6 months until another AF episode. (*C*) Frequent: multiple AF episodes without any 6-month AF-free period. (*D*) Persistent AF: AF lasting continuously for more than 7 days. AT, atrial tachycardia. (An example of a patient without any AF during follow-up is not shown.) (*From* Musat DL, Milstein NS, Pimienta J, Bhatt A, Preminger MW, Sichrovsky TC, Flynn L, Pistilli C, Shaw RE, Mittal S. Incidence, duration, pattern, and burden of de novo atrial arrhythmias detected by continuous ECG monitoring using an implantable loop recorder following ablation of the cavotricuspid isthmus. *Cardiovascular Digital Health Journal* 2020; 1: 114–122; with permission.)

episodes—multiple AF episodes without any 6-month AF-free period; (5) persistent AF—AF lasting continuously for more than 7 days. Whether these patterns affect clinical outcomes, including stroke risk and need for anticoagulation, remains to be defined.

An important area of investigation is the role of continuous ECG monitoring to guide decisions regarding the need for long-term anticoagulation in patients with AF. Current guidelines advocate oral anticoagulation in patients with AF with a CHA_2DS_2-VASc score greater than or equal to 2 in men and greater than or equal to 3 in women.[14] However, it has been shown that incorporation of AF duration further stratifies risk of stroke. The annual stroke risk was greater than 1% in patients with CHA_2DS_2-VASc score greater than or equal to 5 even in the absence of AF, when AF was greater than 6 minutes in duration in patients with CHA_2DS_2-VASc score of 3 or 4, and not until AF was greater than 23.5 hours in patients with CHA_2DS_2-VASc score of 2.[26]

On the other side is using the information to determine the need for anticoagulation following AF ablation. It has been suggested that ILR confirmed absence of AF can be used to safely withhold oral anticoagulation and thus mitigate

bleeding risks inherent to long-term use of oral anticoagulation therapy.[27,28] In the REACT.com study, 59 patients with nonpermanent AF, a $CHADS_2$ score of 1 or 2, who already taking an oral anticoagulant underwent ILR implantation and subsequent daily device interrogation.[27] If there were no AF episodes greater than or equal to 1 hour, oral anticoagulants were discontinued but reinitiated for 30 days following any AF episode greater than or equal to 1 hour. Exposure to anticoagulation was reduced by 94%; importantly, no patient suffered a stroke, suggesting the viability of a "pill-in-the pocket" approach to anticoagulation. A second study enrolled 65 patients with a $CHADS_2$ score of 1 to 3 who had undergone catheter ablation of AF and subsequent ILR implantation.[28] Anticoagulation was then stopped and not resumed unless daily device interrogation showed an episode of AF greater than or equal to 1 hour. Anticoagulation was successfully withheld in 63% of patients; no stroke, transient ischemic attack, or cardioembolic event was observed.

There is a clear desire by patients and physicians to answer the following question: can anticoagulation be stopped in patients with AF in whom catheter ablation has eliminated further episodes of AF. OCEAN is an ongoing study that aims to answer this question.[29] The study is enrolling 1572 patients with AF, a CHA2DS2-VASc score of > 1, who are > 1-year post-successful AF ablation. Patients are randomized to receive either aspirin (75–160 mg) or rivaroxaban (15 mg daily). The primary endpoint is the composite of stroke, systemic embolism, and covert embolic stroke on cerebral emboli over a follow-up duration of 36 months. Unfortunately, this study is not incorporating continuous ECG monitoring, which means that some patients with an apparently successful AF ablation are likely having ongoing AF. Second, the study will not be able to identify patients with a very late recurrence of AF, defined as a first recurrence of AF more than or equal to 1 year after -AF ablation. This phenomenon can be observed in about one-third of patients following AF ablation.[30]

INDICATION-INDEPENDENT CONCERNS

Irrespective of the reason why ECG monitoring with an ILR is initiated in a given patient, there are several important limitations that needs to be addressed.[21] These include battery longevity, ensuring optimal R wave sensing (ideally with P wave sensing as well), accurately differentiating AF from atrial flutter and other forms of organized atrial tachycardias, optimizing the positive predictive value for AF episodes less than 1 hour in duration, reliably transmitting data daily from the ILR to a central Web portal and having a clinical infrastructure to manage the incoming data. In addition, the monthly costs incurred by patients to undergo wireless remote monitoring also need to be better understood and addressed. Overcoming these challenges will ultimately define the role of ILRs for arrhythmia monitoring.

DISCLOSURE

Consultant to Boston Scientific and Medtronic.

REFERENCES

1. Giancatrino S, Lupercio F, Nishimura M, et al. Current and future uses of insertable cardiac monitors. J Am Coll Cardiol EP 2018;4:1383–96.
2. Cheung CC, Krahn AD. Loop recorders for syncope evaluation: what is the evidence? Expert Rev Med Devices 2016;13(11):1021–7.
3. Edvardsson N, Frykman V, Van Mechelen R, et al. On behalf of the PICTURE study investigators. Use of an implantable loop recorder to increase the diagnostic yield in unexplained syncope: results from the PICTURE registry. Europace 2010. https://doi.org/10.1093/europace/euq418.
4. Shen W-K, Sheldon RS, Benditt DG, et al. 2017 ACC/AHA/HRS guideline for the evaluation and management of patients with syncope: a report of the American College of Cardiology/American heart Association Task Force on clinical practice guidelines and the heart rhythm Society. Circulation 2017;136:e60–122.
5. Goldberger ZD, Petek BJ, Brignole M, et al. ACC/AHA/HRS versus ESC guidelines for the diagnosis and management of syncope. J Am Coll Cardiol 2019;74:2410–23.
6. Brignole M, Moya A, de Lange FJ, et al. 2018 ESC Guidelines for the diagnosis and management of syncope. Eur Heart J 2018;39:1883–948.
7. Moya A, Brignole M, Menozzi C, et al. On behalf of the International Study on Syncope of Uncertain Etiology (ISSUE) investigators. Mechanism of syncope in patients with isolated syncope and in patients with tilt-positive syncope. Circulation 2001;104:1261–7.
8. Brignole M, Menozzi C, Moya A, et al. International Study on Syncope of Uncertain Etiology (ISSUE) Investigators. Mechanism of syncope in patients with bundle branch block and negative electrophysiological test. Circulation 2001;104:2045–50.
9. Menozzi C, Brignole M, Garcia-Civera R, et al. On behalf of the International Study on Syncope of Uncertain Etiology (ISSUE) investigators. Mechanism of syncope in patients with heart disease and negative electrophysiologic test. Circulation 2002;105:2741–5.
10. Brignole M, Sutton R, Menozzi C, et al. For the International Study on Syncope of Uncertain Etiology 2 (ISSUE 2) group. Early application of an implantable loop recorder allows effective specific therapy in patients with recurrent suspected neurally mediated syncope. Eur Heart J 2006;27:1085–92.
11. Brignole M, Menozzi C, Moya A, et al. Pacemaker therapy in patients with neurally mediated syncope and documented asystole: third International Study on Syncope of Uncertain Etiology (ISSUE-3): a randomized trial. Circulation 2012;125:2566–71.
12. Hart RG, Sharma M, Mundl H, et al, NAVIGATE ESUS Investigators. Rivaroxaban for stroke prevention after embolic stroke of undetermined source. N Engl J Med 2018;378:2191–201.
13. Diener HC, Sacco RL, Easton JD, et al, RESPECT ESUS Steering Committee Investigators. Dabigatran for prevention of stroke after embolic stroke of undetermined source. N Engl J Med 2019;380:1906_1917.
14. Hindricks G, Potpara T, Dagres N, et al, ESC Scientific Document Group, 2020 ESC Guidelines for the diagnosis and management of atrial fibrillation developed in collaboration with the European Association for Cardio-Thoracic Surgery (EACTS): The Task Force for the diagnosis and management of atrial fibrillation of the European Society of

Cardiology (ESC) Developed with the special contribution of the European Heart Rhythm Association (EHRA) of the ESC. European Heart Journal, ehaa612, https://doi.org/10.1093/eurheartj/ehaa612.

15. Gladstone DJ, Spring M, Dorian P, et al. For the EMRACE investigators and coordinators. Atrial fibrillation in patients with cryptogenic stroke. N Engl J Med 2014;370:2467–77.

16. Sanna T, Diener H-C, Passman RS, et al, for the CRYSTAL AF investigators. Cryptogenic stroke and underlying atrial fibrillation. N Engl J Med 2014; 370:2478–86.

17. Milstein NS, Musat DL, Allred J, et al. Detection of atrial fibrillation using an implantable loop recorder following cryptogenic stroke: implications for post-stroke electrocardiographic monitoring. J Interv Card Electrophysiol 2020;57(1):141–7.

18. Brachmann J, Morillo CA, Sanna T, et al. Uncovering atrial fibrillation beyond short- term monitoring in cryptogenic stroke patients: three-year results from the cryptogenic stroke and underlying atrial fibrillation trial. Circ Arrhythm Electrophysiol 2016;9: e003333.

19. Sawyer LM, Witte KK, Reynolds MR, et al. Cost–effectiveness of an insertable cardiac monitor to detect atrial fibrillation in patients with cryptogenic stroke. J Comp Eff Res 2020. https://doi.org/10.2217/cer-2020-0224.

20. Mittal S, Rogers J, Sankar S, et al. Real-world performance of an enhanced atrial fibrillation detection algorithm in an insertable cardiac monitor. Heart Rhythm 2016;13:1624–30.

21. Lee R, Mittal S. Utility and limitations of long-term monitoring of atrial fibrillation using an implantable loop recorder. Heart Rhythm 2018;15:287–95.

22. Andrade JG, Champagne J, Dubuc M, et al. Khairy, for the CIRCA-DOSE study investigators. Cryoballoon or radiofrequency ablation for atrial fibrillation assessed by continuous monitoring: a randomized clinical trial. Circulation 2019;140:1779–88.

23. Andrade JG, Yao RRJ, Deyell MW, et al. For the CIRCA-DOSE study investigators. Clinical assessment of AF pattern is poorly correlated with AF burden and post ablation outcomes: a CIRCA-DOSE sub-study. J Electrocardiol 2020;60:159–64.

24. Andrade JG, Deyell MW, Verma A, et al. Association of atrial fibrillation episode duration with arrhythmia recurrence following ablation: a secondary analysis of a randomized clinical trial. JAMA Netw Open 2020;3(7):e208748. https://doi.org/10.1001/jamanetworkopen.2020.8748.

25. Musat DL, Milstein NS, Pimienta J, et al. Incidence, duration, pattern, and burden of de novo atrial arrhythmias detected by continuous ECG monitoring using an implantable loop recorder following ablation of the cavotricuspid isthmus. Cardiovasc Digital Health J 2020;1:114–22.

26. Kaplan RM, Koehler J, Ziegler PD, et al. Stroke risk as a function of atrial fibrillation duration and $CHA_2DS_2\text{-}VASc$ score. Circulation 2019;140:1639–46.

27. Passman R, Leong-Sit P, Andrei AC, et al. Targeted anticoagulation for atrial fibrillation guided by continuous rhythm assessment with an insertable cardiac monitor: the Rhythm Evaluation for Anticoagulation with Continuous Monitoring (REACT.COM) pilot study. J Cardiovasc Electrophysiol 2016;27:264–70.

28. Zuern CS, Killias A, Berlitz P, et al. Anticoagulation after catheter ablation of atrial fibrillation guided by implantable cardiac monitors. PACE 2015;38: 688–93.

29. Verma A, Ha ACT, Kirchhof P, et al. The optimal anticoagulation for enhanced-risk patients post-catheter ablation for atrial fibrillation (OCEAN) trial. Am Heart J 2018;197:124–32.

30. Musat DL, Milstein NS, Bhatt A, et al. Incidence and predictors of very late recurrence of atrial fibrillation following cryoballoon pulmonary vein isolation. Circ Arrhythmi Electrophysiol 2020;13:e008646.

Remote Monitoring of Permanent Pacemakers and Implantable Cardioverter Defibrillators

Bryan Wilner, MD, John Rickard, MD, MPH*

KEYWORDS

- Remote monitoring • Remote interrogation • Permanent pacemaker • Cardiac implantable device
- Implantable cardioverter defibrillator

KEY POINTS

- Remote monitoring has been shown to be as safe as routine in-office interrogation for cardiac electronic implantable devices.
- Remote monitoring allows earlier detection of clinically actionable events than in-office device checks.
- Remote monitoring reduces the incidence of inappropriate shocks and allows for earlier detection of atrial fibrillation.
- Remote monitoring may be associated with a reduction in savings on pacemaker and implantable cardioverter defibrillators care, although more data are needed.
- With the easy accessibility and widespread use of smartphones, app-based remote monitoring provides patients with rapid access to their own physiologic data, which may improve compliance with remote monitoring.

HISTORY

The evolution of remote monitoring (RM) of permanent pacemakers and implantable cardioverter defibrillators (ICDs) has paralleled the considerable advancement in the technology of these devices. The first pacemaker was implanted in 1958.[1] Since then, the number of cardiac implantable electronic devices (CIEDs) that have been implanted has grown significantly. In 2006, approximately 280,000 pacemakers and 160,000 ICDs were implanted in North America, with the numbers growing considerably ever since.[2] In 2020, it was estimated that the worldwide number of individuals with ICDs was anywhere between 500,000 and 3 million.[3] The increase in the population of patients with implantable devices has created unique challenges in terms of device follow-up.

Patients with CIEDs traditionally have undergone frequent in-person device interrogations using a dedicated device clinic. With the cardiac device implantation rate increasing as well as the expansion of evidence-based indications for implantation of devices, the demand for in-person device follow-up has spiked, creating an ever-increasing burden on such clinics.[4,5] In addition, studies have shown that patients with CIEDSs have a significant rate of clinical events, such as atrial tachyarrhythmias/atrial fibrillation (AF), that previously were detected only at standard device follow-up visits.[6,7] The advancement in technology of implantable devices has created an ability for

Department of Cardiovascular Medicine, Section of Cardiac Electrophysiology, Heart, Vascular, and Thoracic Institute, Cleveland Clinic, 9500 Euclid Avenue/J2-2, Cleveland, OH 44195, USA
* Corresponding author.
E-mail address: Rickarj2@ccf.org

Card Electrophysiol Clin 13 (2021) 449–457
https://doi.org/10.1016/j.ccep.2021.04.005

RM of devices in which a device can monitor its own function, record arrhythmias and other physiologic parameters, and transmit data to health care providers without the need for frequent in-office checks. RM of these devices has added new challenges to device clinic work flows.[8] With the ability to gather data easily in real time and remotely, RM provides a unique opportunity to improve patient outcomes, identify device malfunctions, and decrease the burden of in-office visits.[9]

RM of CIEDs has undergone tremendous technological advancement since its inception. In 1971, early transtelephonic monitoring (TTM) was developed to monitor the longevity of pacemakers.[10] In the late 1970s and 1980s, its role expanded as a diagnostic tool in which patients had to dial into a central receiving system and manually transmit simple device information. Sensing and capture, battery status, and a real-time electrocardiogram rhythm strip could be generated.[11] Although the use of TTM was shown to reduce the frequency of clinic visits, it did not retrieve diagnostic data from the device, could provide only limited assessment of a pacemaker's function, and had multiple other limitations, such as problems with skin electrode placement and issues related to telephone transmission.[12,13] TTM remained the primary method of RM until relatively recently when home monitors/communicators became available. In the late 1990s, more modern devices started to use inductive technology in which a wand-based radiofrequency platform was used to transfer data wirelessly between a patient's device and a home transceiver. The data then are sent from the transceiver by telephone to a central repository and placed on a secure Web site for the provider to retrieve and review. A prospective analysis with this RM strategy was shown comparable to an in-office device interrogation.[14] Poor patient compliance as well as issues setting up the transmitter at home proved to be hurdles in its inception.[15] In 2001, the first fully automatic platform for RM was released.[16] Transmissions were sent wirelessly at set frequencies to a receiver close to the patient, which then transmitted data to the manufacturer's central source for storage. Data transmitted included tachyarrhythmias, details on shock therapy, physiologic parameters such as heart rate and incidence of arrhythmias, and technical aspects of the leads and generator.

TERMINOLOGY

As defined in the 2015 Heart Rhythm Society (HRS) expert consensus statement on remote interrogation (RI) and RM for cardiovascular implantable electronic devices, it is important to differentiate between the terms RI and RM.[9] RI refers to scheduled remote device interrogations that are intended to reflect in-office checkups.[17] Although the majority of information that would be gathered during an in-office device can be obtained with RI, an important exception is measuring the pacing capture threshold, which is not routinely available on all devices. RM refers to data that are acquired automatically with unscheduled transmissions of any prespecified alerts related to device functioning or to clinical events. Prespecified alerts include changes in lead impedance, development of atrial arrythmias, episodes of ventricular tachycardia or ventricular fibrillation, delivery of shocks, and changes in hemodynamic status.[18,19]

REVIEW OF THE LITERATURE SUPPORTING THE USE OF DEVICES TELEMONITORING

Over the past 2 decades, there has been an explosion of research investigating the clinical utility of RI and RM. In 2004, there were 2 prospective studies that showed that RI was able to provide patient care comparable to an in-office interrogation visit. These studies showed that RIs were safe, provided comprehensive reporting of device function and arrhythmia detection, could be utilized by most patients, and had high patient and clinician satisfaction scores.[14,18] The Pacemaker Remote Follow-up Evaluation and Review (PREFER) clinical trial was the first study to evaluate whether remote pacemaker interrogation could detect clinically actionable events (CAEs) earlier than standard TTM monitoring in 980 patients.[20] CAEs included episodes of atrial tachycardia/AF, ventricular tachycardia, ventricular pacing percentage, changes in atrial or ventricular lead impedance, and battery voltage/elective replacement indicator status. Over a 12-month period, the mean time to first diagnosis of a CAE was earlier in the remote arm than the TTM arm (5.7 months vs 7.7 months, respectively; $P<.0001$). This was one of the first trials validating RM as superior to TTM for managing patients with CIEDs.

In 2008, there was an expert consensus recommendation for regular calendar-based follow-up of 3-month to 6-month checks utilizing either an inpatient visit or RM.[8] RM allows for more rapid detection of clinically significant events compared with conventional follow-up among. The Lumos-T Safety Reduces Routine Office Device Follow-Up (TRUST) clinical trial compared the safety and usefulness of RM in ICD recipients with standard in-clinic follow-up.[21] Over a 1-year follow-up period, it was found that RM allowed for more rapid detection of actionable events compared with conventional monitoring, reduced the number of scheduled and unscheduled hospital evaluations, and demonstrated no increase in all-cause mortality. This was the first trial that showed RM provided continuity of follow-up in a large patient population, allowed continuous surveillance of events requiring immediate attention, and demonstrated the ability to avoid unnecessary in-hospital patient evaluations. RM further was shown to preserve patient retention and adherence to scheduled follow-up compared with in-person evaluation.[22] Several other studies have shown that replacing in-person visits with RM follow-up can decrease the amount of in-person visits in a safe manner and lead to early detection of clinically significant events.[23–25] The Remote Follow-up for ICD-Therapy in Patients Meeting MADIT II Criteria (REFORM) trial found that in prophylactic ICD recipients with automatic daily RM, the extension of the 3-month in-office follow-up interval to 12 months safely reduced the ICD in-person follow-up burden (1.6 vs 3.8 per patient-office visits, respectively; $P<.001$) with no difference in mortality, hospitalization rate, or hospitalization length.[23] The Monitoring Resynchronization Devices and Cardiac Patients (MORE-CARE) trial showed that in patients with advanced heart failure and cardiac resynchronization therapy defibrillators (CRT-Ds), the median delay from device-detected event to clinical decision was shorter in the RM group (2 days vs 29 days, respectively; $P = .004$) compared with the control arm. In addition, in-hospital visits were reduced in the RM arm compared with the control (2 visits/patient/y vs 3.2 visits/patient/y, respectively; $P<.001$).[24] In the Evolution of Management Strategies of Heart Failure Patients with Implantable Defibrillators (EVOLVO) study, RM was shown to reduce emergency department/urgent in-office visits in heart failure patients with an ICD or CRT-D device.[26] The Clinical Evaluation of Remote Notification to Reduce Time to Clinical Decision (CONNECT) trial showed that in patients who underwent ICD insertion, RM with automatic clinician alerts compared with standard in-office follow-up significantly reduced the time to a clinical decision in response to clinical events (4.6 d vs 22 d, respectively; $P<.001$) and was associated with a significant reduction in mean length of hospital stay (3.3 d vs 4 d, respectively; $P = .002$).[25] The Effectiveness and Cost of ICD Follow-Up Schedule with Telecardiology (ECOST) study compared the proportion of major adverse cardiac events (MACEs) in patients who underwent ICD implantation who were assigned to RM versus ambulatory follow-up.[27] Over a follow-up of 24 months, 38.5% of patients

in the RM arm versus 41.5% in the control arm experienced greater than or equal to 1 MACE ($P<.05$), and the overall number of shocks delivered was lower in the RM group compared with the control arm (193 shocks vs 657 shocks, respectively; $P<.05$). Additionally, RM was shown to decrease health care resource utilization. In a nationwide cohort study, it was shown that RM was associated with a 30% reduction in hospitalization costs compared with a non–RM-guided strategy ($8720 mean cost per patient-year vs $12,423 mean cost per patient-year, respectively).[28] In summary, RM has been shown via evidence supported by several randomized clinical trials to detect CAEs earlier, decrease office visits/hospitalizations, and decrease hospital costs compared with in-patient device management. RM was not associated with patient safety concerns compared with traditional in-office checks.

PATIENT AND PHYSICIAN/INSTITUTION RESPONSIBILITIES

Current guidelines give a class I recommendation to using RM as a way to improve patient compliance.[9] Even though there is high-quality evidence to show that RM is associated with superior quality of life[23] and patient convenience,[14] compliance still is a challenge for both patient and caregiver.[29] Successful use of RM begins with physicians and the health care team educating patients about RM and its use as a tool to enhance patient care. Successful use of RM depends on active enrollment of the patient, patient compliance with transmission schedules, and other responsibilities. An observational study reported that among 269,471 patients with automatic RM-capable devices, only 47% of patients were using RM.[30] Barriers to use include lack of cell phone compatibly in early systems, confusion between RM and remote follow-up, language barriers, and inappropriate infrastructure in place for follow-up. Another major barrier to RM use is lack of enrollment. Akar and colleagues[29] identified that among 39,158 patients with newly implanted RM-capable devices, only 62% were RM enrolled and concluded that RM technology is used in less than half of eligible patients. The investigators concluded that the most likely reason for underutilization was lack of enrollment in an RM system.[29] Another barrier to RM is patient participation and compliance. Among patients (n = 118,132) enrolled in an RM system (CareLink [Medtronic, Minneapolis, Minnesota]), overall compliance with RM was 21%. Clinically important predictors of noncompliance include age less than or equal to 40, female sex, smaller clinics, and certain geographic areas.[31] Strategies to improve patient compliance included in-office setup compared with home setup and using an RM patient agreement that is endorsed by the HRS.[32] On the caregiver side, RM requires a complex network in place, including additional staff, the use of the electronic medical record to manage the data, and new work flows to identify important events (such as AF).[33] An optimal organizational model continues to be developed. Midlevel providers, such as nurse practitioners, physician assistants, and nurses trained specifically in RM, can serve as the first contact for RM patients. Such caregivers are tasked with reviewing RM transmissions and collaborating with a supervising physician when required.[34] Even though an optimal organizational model for effective RM varies among different health care organizations (depending on a variety of factors, including the technological limitations of the health system, telecommunication technology, and local infrastructure in place to monitor events), it is imperative for both patient and provider to be actively involved for a successful program.

DISEASE-SPECIFIC MANAGEMENT
Mortality

The effect of RM on all-cause mortality has been studied in several studies. The COMPAS trial was a noninferiority trial that showed no difference in survival in patients with pacemakers randomized to RM versus usual care over an 18-month period ($P = .63$).[35] There are 3 nonrandomized clinical trials that observed a mortality benefit with RM. The ALTITUDE study was a nonrandomized observational study in which patients who received ICD and Cardiac resynchronization therapy (CRT) devices with remote follow-up (n = 69,556) had 1-year and 5-year survival rates that were higher compared with those who received in-office–based follow-up (n = 116,222) (50% reduction; $P<.0001$).[36] A separate observational study evaluated outcomes in 269,471 patients implanted with pacemakers, ICDs, or CRTs with wireless RM and found that survival was better in patients with high adherence to RM (>75% of time in RM) compared with those with both low adherence (<75% of time in RM) and without RM.[30] The EFFECT study was a prospective, nonrandomized study among 987 patients with ICD/CRT-D devices and compared outcomes based on device follow-up strategy.[37] The study concluded that RM is associated with reduced death and cardiovascular hospitalizations compared with standard follow-up.

Overall, the effect of RM on mortality has had mixed results in randomized clinical trials. A major contributing factor to relates to which home monitoring system was used and the percentage of time RM took place. A meta-analysis analyzing 9 clinical trials concluded that RM was comparable with office follow-up in terms of all-cause mortality ($P = .285$).[38] One clinical trial that was included in this meta-analysis—Implant-based Multiparameter Telemonitoring of Patients with Heart Failure (IN-TIME)—did show a significant reduction in all-cause mortality.[39] This study included 665 patients with systolic dysfunction and New York Heart Association (NYHA) functional class II or class IIR symptoms who were assigned randomly to RM or to standard of care. At 1-year follow-up, RM was associated with lower mortality (3.4% in the RM group and 8.7% in the control group; $P = .004$). The RM system used in this study was the Home Monitoring system (Biotronik, Berlin, Germany), which allowed for daily, automatic monitoring transmissions. A meta-analysis of IN-TIME[39] and 2 other randomized clinical trials (ECOST[27] and TRUST[21]) all used the same RM system with daily transmissions (Biotronik Home Monitoring) and found a significant mortality reduction.[40] This is in contrast to 4 other randomized studies that used a different RM platform with less frequent transmissions.[24–26]

Inappropriate Shocks and Shock Reduction

Even though ICDs have been shown to reduce mortality in patients at risk of life-threatening arrhythmias, the fear of experiencing ICD shocks adversely affects patient quality of life.[41,42] Causes of inappropriate shocks include atrial arrhythmias, T-wave oversensing, electromagnetic interference, device malfunction, and lead fracture.[43,44] RM provides an opportunity to recognize device/lead abnormalities and allows for the timely detection and treatment of problems with the goal of decreasing the risk of inappropriate shocks. The ECOST trial showed that among patients randomized to the RM arm, the proportion of appropriate and inappropriate shocks delivered was 71% lower compared with standard in-office follow-up ($P = .02$) and that the number of inappropriate shocks occurred at a 52% lower rate (5% vs 10%, respectively; $P = .03$).[27] All causes of inappropriate shocks (including supraventricular arrhythmias and lead dysfunction) were lower in the RM arm. This also led to increased battery longevity of 7.9 months. Additionally, a prior meta-analysis of 9 randomized clinical trials that compared RM with in-office follow-up showed that RM led to a significant reduction in inappropriate shocks (odds ratio 0.55; $P = .002$).[38] In a retrospective study among 115 patients, RM was shown to reduce the burden of inappropriate shocks related to ICD lead fractures.[45] In summary, RM is associated with a reduction in inappropriate shocks via the timely identification of lead malfunction and supraventricular tachyarrhythmias, offering the potential to start treatment earlier than would have been possible with in-office checks. Such a strategy offers patients a better quality of life and preservation of battery life.

Heart Failure

Heart failure is a major cause of morbidity and mortality worldwide.[46] Over the past 20 years, there has been an increasing number of heart failure patients receiving CIEDs due to trial data documenting improvements in a mortality and hospital admissions in this population.[46,47] The EVOLVO study showed a 35% reduction in urgent admissions and a 21% reduction in urgent follow-up visits for worsening heart failure in the RM arm compared with the control arm.[26] As such, there has been a keen interest to identify factors that predispose to worsening heart failure and ultimately to reduce heart failure admissions and risk of death. RM has the potential to identify patients at risk for worsening heart failure using specific algorithms in the hopes that early intervention can prevent chronic heart failure (CHF) hospitalizations.[48,49] Randomized clinical trials, however, have yielded mixed results. The IN-TIME randomized clinical trial assessed the role of RM among 664 heart failure patients. Over a follow-up of 12 months, automatic daily TM led to a decrease in all-cause mortality (P = .004).[39] This was due to early detection and treatment of ventricular and atrial tachyarrhythmias, early detection of suboptimal device function (eg, recognizing a low percentage of biventricular pacing), and early recognition of symptomatic worsening or noncompliance with medications. In the MORE-CARE study in which heart failure patients with CRT-D were randomized to RM versus in-office follow-up, there was no difference in in mortality or hospitalizations between the 2 arms.[50] In the IN-TIME randomized controlled trial, patients with CHF and an ICD or CRT-D were randomized to RM or standard of care. The primary outcome of all-cause death and hospitalizations was less in the RM arm compared with control (P = .013).

In the clinical trials evaluating the effects of RM in patients with heart failure, sample size, the specific population studied, and the intervention/control groups varied, making direct comparisons somewhat challenging.[48] For example, in the

MORE-CARE study patients had NYHA class III/IV heart failure, compared with IN-TIME in which patients had NYHA class II/III heart failure. Additionally, in the IN-TIME study, RM management was standardized, whereas in MORE-CARE, the RM was based on local clinical practice.

More recently, newer RM-generated data points have been evaluated in terms of identifying patients at high risk for CHF decompensation. For example, transthoracic impedance was shown to correlate inversely with pulmonary capillary wedge pressure, and an alert algorithm based on intrathoracic impedance was developed.[51] In the randomized Diagnostic Outcome Trial in Heart Failure (DOT-HF), patients with CHF who had an ICD or CRT implanted were randomized to an audible alert arm based on impedance versus a control arm. The trial found there was no difference in the primary endpoint of all-cause mortality and hospitalizations.[52] The Remote Management of Heart Failure using Implantable Electronic Devices (REM-HF) trial was a multicenter randomized trial that assigned 1650 patients with heart failure and a CIED to RM or usual care.[53] Parameters measured in the RM arm included arrhythmia burden, biventricular pacing percent, device therapy, impedance, activity level, and device diagnostics. The primary endpoint of death or unplanned hospitalization did not differ between the 2 groups. Several studies combined transthoracic impedance in parallel with other parameters to predict heart failure events. The Program to Access and Review Trending Information and Evaluate Correlation to Symptoms in Patients with Heart Failure (PARTNERS HF) was a prospective observational study among patients with CRT-D. A heart failure device diagnostic algorithm was developed that included AF duration, rapid ventricular rate during AF, heart rate variability, impedance, patient activity, and notable device therapies. Patients with a positive device diagnostic had a 5.5-fold increased risk for heart failure hospitalization within the next month (P<.0001).[54] In the Multisensor Chronic Evaluation in Ambulatory Heart Failure Patients (MULTISENSE), an alert algorithm was developed based on heart sounds, thoracic impedance, heart rate, and activity among patients with CRT-D. The HeartLogic multisensory index and alert algorithm was able to predict impending worsening heart failure events with 70% sensitivity and a median lead time of 34 days before a heart failure event.[55] In summary, through the use of RM, heart failure diagnostic algorithms with increasing sensitivity and specificity have been developed to identify patients at high risk for heart failure hospitalization and other adverse events.

Atrial Fibrillation

AF is well known to increase morbidity and mortality across a wide spectrum of patient populations.[56] RM provides the opportunity for earlier detection of AF and has been shown to have 93% sensitivity in capturing true AF events in the HomeGuide Registry.[34,57,58] Implantable cardiac devices are shown to detect subclinical AF, which is associated with an increased risk of thromboembolic events.[59–62] The risk of thromboembolic events has been shown to rise with increasing duration of AF episodes. In a subgroup of patients from the Mode Selection Trial (MOST), detection of atrial high-rate episodes lasting more than 5 minutes detected through RM was associated with a 2-fold increase in the risk of death or stroke.[63,64] The TRENDS study found that AT/AF burden greater than or equal to 5.5 hours was associated with an approximate doubling of the risk of thromboembolic events.[60] It has been suggested that in patients with AF episodes, risk stratification for thromboembolic events can be improved by combining $CHADS_2$ score with AF presence and duration.[61] In summary, RM allows for the early identification and duration of subclinical AF, which ultimately can help guide treatment strategies.

Guidelines

The HRS published an expert consensus statement on RI and RM for cardiovascular implantable electronic devices in 2015.[9] The class I recommendations for device and disease management include the following: (1) RM should be performed for surveillance of lead function and battery conservation; (2) patients with a CIED component that has been recalled or is on advisory should be enrolled in RM to enable early detection of actionable events; (3) RM is useful to reduce the incidence of inappropriate ICD shocks; and (4) RM is useful for the early detection and quantification of AF.

Class I recommendations for device follow-up include the following: (1) Implementation of a strategy for remote CIED monitoring and Interrogation, combined with at minimum annual in-person evaluation; (2) all patients with CIEDs should be offered RM; (3) patients should be educated about RM, responsibilities, and expectations; (3) all cardiac implanted devices be checked through direct patient contact 2 weeks to 12 weeks after implantation; (4) health care professionals responsible for interpreting RM transmissions must have the same qualifications as those performing in clinic assessments; and (5) RM programs should develop and document appropriate policies and procedures to govern program operations.

FUTURE DIRECTIONS

In the current era of digital health, in which there is widespread use of smartphones, there are a lot of exciting uses of app-based RM that potentially could improve patient care and outcomes. For example, new, fully automated app-based systems have been developed, which, once downloaded onto a patient's smartphone, are able to download information from the pacemaker/ICD and transmit such data to a network via cellular networks. Data that are transmitted include events related to lead impedance, low battery voltage, atrial arrhythmia burden, ventricular tachycardia episodes, fast ventricular rates during atrial tachycardia/AF, capture management, and percentage of ventricular pacing. Such technology allows patients to access their own data rapidly. Recently, the prospective observational BlueSync Field Evaluation study evaluated the use of a smartphone-based app. Preliminary data demonstrated that patients who used the mobile app were more likely to adhere to their RM schedule than patients who used traditional bedside monitors.[65] Other future uses of RM include wireless programming of devices, although security concerns over this may be a barrier.

CLINICS CARE POINTS

- RM has been shown to be as safe as routine in-office interrogation for CIEDs.
- RM allows for earlier detection of CAEs than in-office device interrogation.
- RM reduces the incidence of inappropriate shocks.
- RM allows for earlier detection of AF.
- App-based RM with smartphones provides patients with rapid access to their own cardiac data, which may improve compliance with RM.

DISCLOSURE

The authors have nothing to disclose.

REFERENCES

1. Aquilina O. A brief history of cardiac pacing. Images Paediatr Cardiol 2006;8(2):17–81.

2. Eucomed. [EUCOMED (European Medical Technology Industry Association]. Available at: http://www.eucomed.be/. Accessed November 11, 2020.

3. Puette JA, Malek R, Ellison MB. Pacemaker. StatPearls. Treasure Island (FL): StatPearls Publishing Copyright © 2020, StatPearls Publishing LLC; 2020.

4. Gregoratos G, Abrams J, Epstein AE, et al. ACC/AHA/NASPE 2002 guideline update for implantation of cardiac pacemakers and antiarrhythmia devices: summary article: a report of the American College of Cardiology/American Heart Association Task Force on Practice Guidelines (ACC/AHA/NASPE Committee to Update the 1998 Pacemaker Guidelines). Circulation 2002;106(16):2145–61.

5. Epstein AE, DiMarco JP, Ellenbogen KA, et al. ACC/AHA/HRS 2008 Guidelines for Device-Based Therapy of Cardiac Rhythm Abnormalities: a report of the American College of Cardiology/American Heart Association Task Force on Practice Guidelines (Writing Committee to Revise the ACC/AHA/NASPE 2002 Guideline Update for Implantation of Cardiac Pacemakers and Antiarrhythmia Devices) developed in collaboration with the American Association for Thoracic Surgery and Society of Thoracic Surgeons. J Am Coll Cardiol 2008; 51(21):e1–62.

6. Orlov MV, Ghali JK, Araghi-Niknam M, et al. Asymptomatic atrial fibrillation in pacemaker recipients: incidence, progression, and determinants based on the atrial high rate trial. Pacing Clin Electrophysiol 2007;30(3):404–11.

7. Ghali JK, Orlov MV, Araghi-Niknam M, et al. The influence of symptoms and device detected atrial tachyarrhythmias on medical management: insights from A-HIRATE. Pacing Clin Electrophysiol 2007; 30(7):850–7.

8. Wilkoff BL, Auricchio A, Brugada J, et al. HRS/EHRA expert consensus on the monitoring of cardiovascular implantable electronic devices (CIEDs): description of techniques, indications, personnel, frequency and ethical considerations. Heart Rhythm 2008;5(6): 907–25.

9. Slotwiner D, Varma N, Akar JG, et al. HRS expert consensus statement on remote interrogation and monitoring for cardiovascular implantable electronic devices. Heart Rhythm 2015;12(7):e69–100.

10. Furman S, Escher DJ. Transtelephone pacemaker monitoring: five years later. Ann Thorac Surg 1975; 20(3):326–38.

11. Griffin JC, Schuenemeyer TD, Hess KR, et al. Pacemaker follow-up: its role in the detection and correction of pacemaker system malfunction. Pacing Clin Electrophysiol 1986;9(3):387–91.

12. Schoenfeld MH. Follow-up of the paced patient. 2nd edition. Philadelphia, PA: Clinical Cardiac Pacing and Defibrillation; 2000. p. 895–929.

13. Dressing T, Schott R, McDowell C, et al. Transtelephonic ICD follow-up is better: more comprehensive, less intrusive, and more desirable. (abstract) PACE 2002;25:219.

14. Schoenfeld MH, Compton SJ, Mead RH, et al. Remote monitoring of implantable cardioverter defibrillators: a prospective analysis. Pacing Clin Electrophysiol 2004;27(6 Pt 1):757–63.

15. Cronin EM, Ching EA, Varma N, et al. Remote monitoring of cardiovascular devices: a time and activity analysis. Heart Rhythm 2012;9(12):1947–51.

16. Theuns DA, Res JC, Jordaens LJ. Home monitoring in ICD therapy: future perspectives. Europace 2003; 5(2):139–42.

17. Burri H. Remote follow-up and continuous remote monitoring, distinguished. Europace 2013;15(Suppl 1):i14–6.

18. Joseph GK, Wilkoff BL, Dresing T, et al. Remote interrogation and monitoring of implantable cardioverter defibrillators. J Interv Card Electrophysiol 2004;11(2):161–6.

19. Ricci RP, Morichelli L, Santini M. Home monitoring remote control of pacemaker and implantable cardioverter defibrillator patients in clinical practice: impact on medical management and health-care resource utilization. Europace 2008;10(2):164–70.

20. Crossley GH, Chen J, Choucair W, et al. Clinical benefits of remote versus transtelephonic monitoring of implanted pacemakers. J Am Coll Cardiol 2009; 54(22):2012–9.

21. Varma N, Epstein AE, Irimpen A, et al. Efficacy and safety of automatic remote monitoring for implantable cardioverter-defibrillator follow-up: the Lumos-T Safely Reduces Routine Office Device Follow-up (TRUST) trial. Circulation 2010;122(4):325–32.

22. Varma N, Michalski J, Stambler B, et al. Superiority of automatic remote monitoring compared with in-person evaluation for scheduled ICD follow-up in the TRUST trial - testing execution of the recommendations. Eur Heart J 2014;35(20):1345–52.

23. Hindricks G, Elsner C, Piorkowski C, et al. Quarterly vs. yearly clinical follow-up of remotely monitored recipients of prophylactic implantable cardioverter-defibrillators: results of the REFORM trial. Eur Heart J 2014;35(2):98–105.

24. Boriani G, Da Costa A, Ricci RP, et al. The MOnitoring Resynchronization dEvices and CARdiac patiEnts (MORE-CARE) randomized controlled trial: phase 1 results on dynamics of early intervention with remote monitoring. J Med Internet Res 2013; 15(8):e167.

25. Crossley GH, Boyle A, Vitense H, et al. The CONNECT (Clinical Evaluation of Remote Notification to Reduce Time to Clinical Decision) trial: the value of wireless remote monitoring with automatic clinician alerts. J Am Coll Cardiol 2011;57(10):1181–9.

26. Landolina M, Perego GB, Lunati M, et al. Remote monitoring reduces healthcare use and improves quality of care in heart failure patients with implantable defibrillators: the evolution of management strategies of heart failure patients with implantable defibrillators (EVOLVO) study. Circulation 2012; 125(24):2985–92.

27. Guédon-Moreau L, Lacroix D, Sadoul N, et al. A randomized study of remote follow-up of implantable cardioverter defibrillators: safety and efficacy report of the ECOST trial. Eur Heart J 2013;34(8):605–14.

28. Piccini JP, Mittal S, Snell J, et al. Impact of remote monitoring on clinical events and associated health care utilization: a nationwide assessment. Heart Rhythm 2016;13(12):2279–86.

29. Akar JG, Bao H, Jones P, et al. Use of remote monitoring of newly implanted cardioverter-defibrillators: insights from the patient related determinants of ICD remote monitoring (PREDICT RM) study. Circulation 2013;128(22):2372–83.

30. Varma N, Piccini JP, Snell J, et al. The relationship between level of adherence to automatic wireless remote monitoring and survival in pacemaker and defibrillator patients. J Am Coll Cardiol 2015; 65(24):2601–10.

31. Rosenfeld LE, Patel AS, Ajmani VB, et al. Compliance with remote monitoring of ICDS/CRTDS in a real-world population. Pacing Clin Electrophysiol 2014;37(7):820–7.

32. Ren X, Apostolakos C, Vo TH, et al. Remote monitoring of implantable pacemakers: in-office setup significantly improves successful data transmission. Clin Cardiol 2013;36(10):634–7.

33. Mittal S, Movsowitz C, Varma N. The modern EP practice: EHR and remote monitoring. Cardiol Clin 2014;32(2):239–52.

34. Ricci RP, Morichelli L, D'Onofrio A, et al. Effectiveness of remote monitoring of CIEDs in detection and treatment of clinical and device-related cardiovascular events in daily practice: the HomeGuide Registry. Europace 2013;15(7):970–7.

35. Mabo P, Victor F, Bazin P, et al. A randomized trial of long-term remote monitoring of pacemaker recipients (the COMPAS trial). Eur Heart J 2012;33(9): 1105–11.

36. Saxon LA, Hayes DL, Gilliam FR, et al. Long-term outcome after ICD and CRT implantation and influence of remote device follow-up: the ALTITUDE survival study. Circulation 2010;122(23):2359–67.

37. De Simone A, Leoni L, Luzi M, et al. Remote monitoring improves outcome after ICD implantation: the clinical efficacy in the management of heart failure (EFFECT) study. Europace 2015;17(8):1267–75.

38. Parthiban N, Esterman A, Mahajan R, et al. Remote monitoring of implantable cardioverter-defibrillators: a systematic review and meta-analysis of clinical outcomes. J Am Coll Cardiol 2015;65(24):2591–600.

39. Hindricks G, Taborsky M, Glikson M, et al. Implant-based multiparameter telemonitoring of patients with heart failure (IN-TIME): a randomised controlled trial. Lancet 2014;384(9943):583–90.

40. Hindricks G, Varma N, Kacet S, et al. Daily remote monitoring of implantable cardioverter-defibrillators: insights from the pooled patient-level data from three randomized controlled trials (IN-TIME, ECOST, TRUST). Eur Heart J 2017;38(22):1749–55.

41. Moss AJ, Greenberg H, Case RB, et al. Long-term clinical course of patients after termination of ventricular tachyarrhythmia by an implanted defibrillator. Circulation 2004;110(25):3760–5.

42. Sears SF, Rosman L, Sasaki S, et al. Defibrillator shocks and their effect on objective and subjective patient outcomes: results of the PainFree SST clinical trial. Heart Rhythm 2018;15(5):734–40.

43. Kulkarni N, Link MS. Causes and prevention of inappropriate implantable cardioverter-defibrillator shocks. Card Electrophysiol Clin 2018;10(1):67–74.

44. van Rees JB, Borleffs CJ, de Bie MK, et al. Inappropriate implantable cardioverter-defibrillator shocks: incidence, predictors, and impact on mortality. J Am Coll Cardiol 2011;57(5):556–62.

45. Souissi Z, Guédon-Moreau L, Boulé S, et al. Impact of remote monitoring on reducing the burden of inappropriate shocks related to implantable cardioverter-defibrillator lead fractures: insights from a French single-centre registry. Europace 2016;18(6):820–7.

46. Yancy CW, Jessup M, Bozkurt B, et al. 2013 ACCF/AHA guideline for the management of heart failure: executive summary: a report of the American College of Cardiology Foundation/American Heart Association Task Force on practice guidelines. Circulation 2013;128(16):1810–52.

47. Bardy GH, Lee KL, Mark DB, et al. Amiodarone or an implantable cardioverter-defibrillator for congestive heart failure. N Engl J Med 2005;352(3):225–37.

48. Hawkins NM, Virani SA, Sperrin M, et al. Predicting heart failure decompensation using cardiac implantable electronic devices: a review of practices and challenges. Eur J Heart Fail 2016;18(8):977–86.

49. Vollmann D, Nägele H, Schauerte P, et al. Clinical utility of intrathoracic impedance monitoring to alert patients with an implanted device of deteriorating chronic heart failure. Eur Heart J 2007;28(15): 1835–40.

50. Boriani G, Da Costa A, Quesada A, et al. Effects of remote monitoring on clinical outcomes and use of healthcare resources in heart failure patients with biventricular defibrillators: results of the MORE-CARE multicentre randomized controlled trial. Eur J Heart Fail 2017;19(3):416–25.

51. Yu CM, Wang L, Chau E, et al. Intrathoracic impedance monitoring in patients with heart failure: correlation with fluid status and feasibility of early warning
preceding hospitalization. Circulation 2005;112(6):
841–8.

52. van Veldhuisen DJ, Braunschweig F, Conraads V,
et al. Intrathoracic impedance monitoring, audible
patient alerts, and outcome in patients with heart
failure. Circulation 2011;124(16):1719–26.

53. Morgan JM, Kitt S, Gill J, et al. Remote management
of heart failure using implantable electronic devices.
Eur Heart J 2017;38(30):2352–60.

54. Whellan DJ, Ousdigian KT, Al-Khatib SM, et al. Combined heart failure device diagnostics identify patients at higher risk of subsequent heart failure
hospitalizations: results from PARTNERS HF (Program to Access and Review Trending Information
and Evaluate Correlation to Symptoms in Patients
with Heart Failure) study. J Am Coll Cardiol 2010;
55(17):1803–10.

55. Boehmer JP, Hariharan R, Devecchi FG, et al.
A multisensor algorithm predicts heart failure events
in patients with implanted devices: results from the
MultiSENSE study. JACC Heart Fail 2017;5(3):
216–25.

56. Benjamin EJ, Wolf PA, D'Agostino RB, et al. Impact
of atrial fibrillation on the risk of death: the Framingham Heart Study. Circulation 1998;98(10):946–52.

57. Varma N, Stambler B, Chun S. Detection of atrial
fibrillation by implanted devices with wireless data
transmission capability. Pacing Clin Electrophysiol
2005;28(Suppl 1):S133–6.

58. Ricci RP, Morichelli L, Santini M. Remote control of
implanted devices through Home Monitoring

technology improves detection and clinical management of atrial fibrillation. Europace 2009;11(1):
54–61.

59. Healey JS, Connolly SJ, Gold MR, et al. Subclinical
atrial fibrillation and the risk of stroke. N Engl J
Med 2012;366(2):120–9.

60. Glotzer TV, Daoud EG, Wyse DG, et al. The relationship between daily atrial tachyarrhythmia burden
from implantable device diagnostics and stroke
risk: the TRENDS study. Circ Arrhythm Electrophysiol 2009;2(5):474–80.

61. Botto GL, Padeletti L, Santini M, et al. Presence and
duration of atrial fibrillation detected by continuous
monitoring: crucial implications for the risk of thromboembolic events. J Cardiovasc Electrophysiol
2009;20(3):241–8.

62. Capucci A, Santini M, Padeletti L, et al. Monitored
atrial fibrillation duration predicts arterial embolic
events in patients suffering from bradycardia and
atrial fibrillation implanted with antitachycardia
pacemakers. J Am Coll Cardiol 2005;46(10):
1913–20.

63. Glotzer TV, Hellkamp AS, Zimmerman J, et al. Atrial
high rate episodes detected by pacemaker diagnostics predict death and stroke: report of the Atrial
Diagnostics Ancillary Study of the MOde Selection
Trial (MOST). Circulation 2003;107(12):1614–9.

64. Holtzman JN, Wadhera RK, Choi E, et al. Trends in
utilization and spending on remote monitoring of
pacemakers and implantable cardioverter-
defibrillators among Medicare beneficiaries. Heart
Rhythm 2020;17(11):1917–21.

65. New Data Unveiled at Heart Rhythm 2020 Demonstrate Effectiveness of App-Based Remote Monitoring of Medtronic Cardiac Devices. 2020.

Current Guidelines and Clinical Practice

Charles J. Love, MD

KEYWORDS

- Arrhythmia monitoring guidelines • Guidelines • Ambulatory cardiac monitoring
- Arrhythmia evaluation

KEY POINTS

- Indications and guidelines trail technology, and reimbursement trails guidelines.
- Generally, guidelines from different organizations parallel each other; however, there are some differences based on geography.
- Choice of monitoring modality should be based on the duration and frequency of the episodes, as well as the degree of symptoms and ability of the patient to respond to the event.

OVERVIEW

Guidelines for choosing and billing for different types of monitoring methods vary widely around the world. However, there have been recent documents developed jointly by the major heart rhythm and heart societies regarding indications and use of the different modalities. As these technologies continue to evolve and to become more available, challenges regarding what to use and whether one can get reimbursed for prescribing a particular modality are constantly evolving. The sequence of product development, studies showing efficacy, regulatory agency approval, and subsequent approval for payment by government and private payers takes years. Just because a new product is introduced and shows efficacy does not guarantee that there will be reimbursement. However, it is clear that remote and home monitoring of cardiac implantable electronic devices (CIEDs) provides earlier detection of arrhythmias compared with periodic office device interrogation of devices.

In 2017, guidelines were published regarding the evaluation of syncope.[1] Within this guideline, there is a class 1 (C-EO) recommendation stating "The choice of a specific cardiac monitor should be determined on the basis of the frequency and nature of syncope events. The technology of cardiac rhythm monitoring is dynamic and advancing at rapid speed...Their selection and usefulness are highly dependent on patient characteristics with regard to the frequency of syncope and the likelihood of an arrhythmic cause of syncope." This recommendation provides a very general approach to which type of technology one should choose to evaluate a particular patient. For example, a patient that has a syncopal event once every 6 months would not likely benefit from 24-hour monitoring, whereas a patient that has multiple daily symptoms of palpitations should not have a subcutaneous cardiac rhythm monitor (SCRM) placed. An excellent overview of the different options and their strengths is shown in **Table 1** as published in the ISHINE-Heart Rhythm Association (HRS) consensus statement in 2017 (see **Table 1**; **Table 2**).[2]

A new class of heart rhythm monitoring devices IS the smartphones and wearables. These devices are not useful for asymptomatic patients, for patients having very short episodes, or for patients that become incapacitated at the time of their event. They are also not useful for patients that cannot manage the technology, as it requires one to be able to acquire and transmit the heart rhythm strips manually. However, for adept patients experiencing longer episodes of symptoms, such as palpitations or lightheadedness, this technology can provide an inexpensive and long-term solution. A challenge for the health care provider is that of being overwhelmed with patient

Johns Hopkins Hospital, 600 N. Wolfe St / Carnegie 584, Baltimore, MD 21287, USA
E-mail address: cjlovemd@gmail.com

Card Electrophysiol Clin 13 (2021) 459–471
https://doi.org/10.1016/j.ccep.2021.05.003
1877-9182/21/© 2021 Elsevier Inc. All rights reserved.

Table 1
Characteristics of ambulatory cardiac monitoring devices

Duration of Recording	<1 min	24–48 h	3–7 d	1–4 wk	≤36 mo
Types of recorder	External event recorder Smartphone-based recorder	Standard Holter recorder Mobile cardiac telemetry	Patch/vest/belt recorder Mobile cardiac telemetry Event loop recorder	Patch/vest/belt recorder External loop recorder Mobile cardiac telemetry	Implantable loop recorder
Modality of recording					
Event recording	✔	✔	✔	✔	✔
Continuous recording		✔	✔	✔	✔
Autotrigger recording			✔	✔	
Number of recording leads					
1 lead (2 electrodes)	✔	✔	✔	✔	✔
2 leads (3 electrodes)		✔	✔	✔	
3 leads (5–7 electrodes)		✔	✔	✔	
12 leads (10 electrodes)		✔			
Type of recording system					
Adhesive wired electrodes		✔	✔	✔	
Patch/vest/belt wireless system			✔	✔	✔
Built-in electrodes	✔				✔
Available analyses					
Arrhythmia analysis	✔	✔	✔	✔	
ST analysis		✔	✔	✔	
Heart rate variability		✔	✔	✔	
QT dynamicity		✔	✔	✔	
Heart rate turbulence		✔	✔	✔	
Holter-derived respiration		✔	✔	✔	
QRS late potentials		✔			
P-wave averaging		✔			
T-wave variability		✔			
Activity level		✔	✔	✔	

Frequency of symptoms should dictate the type of recording: longer-term ECG monitoring is required for more infrequent events. Correlation of (or lack of) symptoms and arrhythmias is key. The most appropriate clinical workflow may include a continuous (short-term 24 h and up to 7 d) AECG monitoring, which if unsuccessful, is followed by intermittent external loop recording (long-term from weeks to months). For those patients remaining undiagnosed after prolonged noninvasive monitoring, ILR may be necessary.

From Steinberg JS, Varma NJ, Cygankiewicz I, et. Al. 2017 ISHNE-HRS expert consensus statement on ambulatory ECG and external cardiacmonitoring/telemetry. Heart Rhythm 2017;14:e55–e96 (International Society for Holter and Noninvasive Electrocardiology); with permission.

Table 2
Advantages and major limitations of AECG techniques

ECG Monitoring Technique	Advantages	Limitations
Holter monitoring	• Ability to record and document continuous 3- to 12-lead ECG signal simultaneously with a variety of other biological signals during normal daily activities • Familiarity of physicians with analysis software programs and a wide availability of third-party scanning services that outsource the equipment and generate preliminary diagnostic reports	• Frequent noncompliance with symptom logs and event markers • Frequent electrode detachments • Signal quality issues due to skin adherence artifacts, wire entanglements, and occasional skin dermatitis caused by electrode gels • Absence of real-time data analysis • Poor patient acceptance of wire-electrode systems
Patch ECG monitors	• Long-term recording of 14 d or longer • Excellent patient acceptance	• Records a limited ECG from closely spaced electrodes comprising a time series of P-, Q-, R-, ST-, and T-wave sequence with lower-voltage amplitudes without information on their spatial orientation, thus lacking localization ability of arrhythmia origin • Inconsistent optimal ECG signal quality due to varying body types
External loop recorders	• Records only selected ECG segments of fixed duration marked as events either automatically or manually by the patient • Immediate alarm generation upon event detection	• Records a single-lead ECG sequence without information on spatial orientation of P, Q, R, ST, and T waves, thus lacking localization ability of arrhythmia origin; P waves may not be visible • No capability to continuously document cardiac rhythm • Requires patients to wear electrodes continuously during the recording period
Event recorders	• Records only selected ECG segments of fixed duration after an event is detected by the patient • Immediate alarm generation upon the event detection	• Single-lead devices do not indicate the origin of many arrhythmias • No capability to continuously document cardiac rhythm

(continued on next page)

Table 2
(continued)

ECG Monitoring Technique	Advantages	Limitations
	• Well tolerated by the patient	• Diagnostic yield of event recorders is highly dependent on patient's ability to recognize correct symptom
Mobile cardiac telemetry (MCT)	• Multilead MCT devices can record pseudo-standard, 3-lead ECG, hence has a much higher sensitivity and specificity of arrhythmia detection as compared with single-lead devices • Can stream the data continuously to caregivers; often combines the functionality of traditional 3-lead Holter event and loop recorder, for example, programmed to autodetect and autosend events at certain times (eg, 1 every 10 min) • Immediate alarm generation upon an event detection without patient interaction or manual activation	• Electrode-wire MCT devices require daily electrode changes, and thus, patient acceptance is reduced for long-term monitoring applications

From Steinberg JS, Varma NJ, Cygankiewicz I, et. Al. 2017 ISHNE-HRS expert consensus statement on ambulatory ECG and external cardiacmonitoring/telemetry. Heart Rhythm 2017;14:e55–e96 (International Society for Holter and Noninvasive Electrocardiology); with permission.

transmissions, as well as the lack of reimbursement for reviewing the strips, and this is a case of the technology being available without guidelines for reimbursement from the payers.

In the 2018 American College of Cardiology/American Heart Association (ACC/AHA)/HRS guideline on the evaluation and management of patients with bradycardia and cardiac conduction delay,[3] wearables are designated as class 2, stating they "…may provide diagnostic data that contribute to disease detection and management when integrated into the clinical context and physician judgement."

With regard to other modalities, the same document recommended the use of ambulatory electrocardiographic (ECG) monitoring, Holter, extended Holter, mobile cardiac telemetry monitoring as follows:

1. Holter: Symptoms frequent enough to be detected within the monitoring period (24–72 hours, but longer now with new technology)
2. Event monitors (ie, patient activated): Not as useful in asymptomatic patients or those with incapacitating symptoms
3. External loop recorders (patient or automatically triggered): Symptoms likely to occur during monitoring period of 2 to 6 weeks. May be symptomatic (patient triggered) or have an automatic trigger
4. External patch recorders: Single-lead recording (leadless), patient/autotrigger, 2 to 14 days, good for atrial fibrillation (AF) burden
5. Mobile cardiac outpatient telemetry (MCOT): Up to 30 days, preprogrammed arrythmia detection or patient activated, autotransmitted 24/7 to attended monitoring station, good for high-risk patients needing real-time monitoring, best for brief, subtle, or infrequent episodes
6. Implantable loop recorder (ILR)/SCRM: Patient or autotrigger. Recurrent, infrequent, unexplained symptoms with or without structural heart disease. In addition, these were designated as class IIa (C-LC). They are recommended for patients with infrequent symptoms (30 days between symptoms) suspected to be caused by bradycardia. Long-term ambulatory monitoring with an implantable cardiac monitor is reasonable if initial noninvasive evaluation is nondiagnostic.

Further guidelines regarding the use of ILR/ SCRMs are discussed in the HRS Expert

Consensus Statement on remote interrogation and monitoring for cardiovascular implantable electronic devices *Heart Rhythm* published in 2015.[4] Here, it is discussed how these devices "play an important role in detecting infrequent arrhythmias and evaluating syncope." They are especially useful to diagnose occult AF as a cause of cryptogenic stroke. Although they do cite 2 studies suggesting that ILR/SCRMs may be useful in conjunction with implantable cardioverter defibrillators, this is a situation whereby professional society guidelines lag behind the science, with reimbursement guidelines nonexistent.

IMPLANTABLE LOOP RECORDER GUIDELINES BASED ON THE CURRENT HEART RHYTHM ASSOCIATION DOCUMENT

Class I: An ILR is indicated in the evaluation of patients with infrequent recurrent syncope of uncertain origin, especially when ambulatory monitoring is inconclusive.

Class 1: An ILR is indicated in patients with syncope and high-risk criteria in whom a comprehensive evaluation did not demonstrate a cause of syncope or lead to a specific treatment, and who do not have conventional indications for primary prevention implantable cardioverter-defibrillator (ICD) or pacemaker.

Class 2: An ILR can be considered in patients with palpitations, dizziness, presyncope, and frequent premature ventricular complexes (PVCs)/nonsustained ventricular tachycardia (VT), and in those with suspected AF, and following AF ablation.

Interestingly, as opposed to the HRS guidelines, the European Heart Rhythm Association (EHRA) guidelines[5] state the following:

Class 2: Outside of the research context patients with cryptogenic stroke may not receive an ILR.

SYNCOPE

The effectiveness of any cardiac monitoring strategy to diagnose the cause of syncope as related to the frequency of the events and the duration of monitoring. Other factors to consider are the presence and duration of any prodrome, and how quickly the patient becomes unconscious. If patient activation is required and the event is sudden, there may not be an opportunity for triggering of the device. Events that happen infrequently are unlikely to be diagnosed with standard external recording monitors. Conversely, there is no need to implant a loop recorder into a patient who is having daily events. The newest generation of patch recorders offers up to 1 month of monitoring and is generally well tolerated and accepted by patients. For patients that require continuous observation during the monitoring period, MCOT is an excellent option.

Based on general principles, the choice of which type of monitoring to prescribe is based on the clinical situation and tolerance of the patient for any particular strategy. The guidelines leave a great deal of latitude to the clinician to decide which modality to choose[1]:

Class IIa(B-NR): To evaluate selected ambulatory patients with syncope of suspected arrhythmic cause, the following external cardiac monitoring approaches can be useful:

1. Holter monitor
2. Transtelephonic monitor
3. External loop recorder
4. Patch recorder
5. MCOT

CRYPTOGENIC STROKE, ATRIAL FIBRILLATION

The multisociety 2020 guidelines[6] regarding the use of ILRs relative to diagnosing and managing AF state the following:

Class 1: AF is more likely to be detected after cryptogenic stroke with more intense investigation with longer and more sophisticated monitoring.

Class 1: Long-term ECG monitoring techniques, such as transtelephonic ECG monitoring or cardiac event recorders or ILR, can increase yield of AF diagnosis after cryptogenic stroke in selected patients.

Class 1: The use of an ILR should be considered for detecting AF in selected patients who are at higher risk of AF development, including the elderly, and patients with cardiovascular risk factors or comorbidities.

However, the AF guidelines[7] classifies the use of ILR differently:

Class 2a(B-R): In patients with cryptogenic stroke (ie, stroke of unknown cause) in whom external ambulatory monitoring is inconclusive, implantation of a cardiac monitor (loop recorder) is reasonable to optimize detection of silent AF.

The 2016 European Society of Cardiology (ESC) guidelines[8] recommend screening for AF by pulse taking or ECG rhythm strip in patients older than 65 years of age as class I(B). However, in higher-risk patients, the guidelines are as follows:

Class 1(A): In patients with transient ischemic attack or ischemic stroke, screening for AF is recommended by short-term ECG recording followed by continuous ECG monitoring for at least 72 hours.

Class 1: Serial Holter monitoring may be considered if longer-duration monitoring tools are not available.

Class 1(B): Interrogation if CIEDs on a regular basis for atrial high rate episodes (AHRE).

Class 1(B): Patients with AHRE should undergo further ECG monitoring to document AF before initiating AF therapy (if intracardiac electrograms are not diagnostic).

Class 2a(B): In stroke patients, additional ECG monitoring by long-term noninvasive ECG monitors or ILR should be considered to document silent AF.

Class 2a(B): Systematic ECG screening may be considered to detect AF in patients aged older than 75 years, or those at high stroke risk.

EHRA adds the following[5]:

Class 2: Holter monitoring may be considered for detection of occult AF in high-risk patients who have no CIEDs and have no indication for long-term event monitoring.

Class 2: Holter monitoring may be used as a "step-in" screening strategy or in combination with other screening tools to improve detection of subclinical arrhythmia and to select candidates for long-term monitoring.

More challenging is dealing with data accumulated by implanted pacemakers and ICDs. These devices frequently find episodes of nonsustained AF and other arrhythmias. Current recommendations[7] for managing these patients make it unclear as to how to manage many of the shorter-term events detected, even though it is apparent that there is an incremental risk of thromboembolic events based on the duration of the arrhythmia. The results of prospective trials are awaited to answer the question of how to manage these patients. These guidelines suggest the following:

Class 1 (B-NR): In patients with CIEDs (pacemakers or ICD), the presence of recorded atrial high-rate episodes (AHREs) should prompt further evaluation to document clinically relevant AF to guide treatment decisions.

ASSESSMENT OF PREMATURE VENTRICULAR COMPLEX BURDEN

PVCs may be associated directly with symptoms or may induce a strain-related cardiomyopathy.

Current guidelines for assessing these are based on the multisociety recommendations[2,6] and do not specify a specific monitoring strategy. However, these data may be obtained by any continuous, noninvasive monitoring modality unless an implantable device is already present to accumulate the data. ILRs are NOT particularly useful for this purpose, as they are currently not able to differentiate heart beats based on QRS morphology, but only by whether they are regular or irregular. Dual-chamber CIEDs are good at measuring PVC burden (as defined by 2 ventricular events without an interceding atrial event).

Class 1: Periodic monitoring of PVC burden (every 6 months) and left ventricular ejection fraction (LVEF) and dimensions are useful in patients with frequent, asymptomatic PVCs and a normal LVEF and dimensions.

Class 1: PVC burden exceeding 20% is associated with a higher risk of PVC-related cardiomyopathy.

Class 1: PVC burden lower than 10% is associated with a lower risk of PVC-related cardiomyopathy.

Class 1: An evaluation of cardiac function and screening for heart failure symptoms should be considered in patients with frequent ventricular ectopy (>10,000 PVCs within 24 hours or 10% of the QRS complexes over a more extended timeframe).

Class 1: An evaluation of cardiac function and screening for heart failure symptoms may be considered in patients with frequent multiform PVCs, PVCs with a QRS duration of 150 milliseconds, or PVCs with a coupling interval of ≥450 milliseconds.

REMOTE MONITORING OF CARDIAC IMPLANTABLE ELECTRONIC DEVICES

Guidelines for remote monitoring of CIEDs in general were published in 2015.[4] The basis for remote monitoring is to detect clinically significant arrhythmias (eg, occult AF, AF with rapid ventricular response, ventricular arrhythmias), as well as system abnormalities (eg, battery depletion, lead fracture, circuit failure) before they become clinically significant. Early intervention for newly diagnosed AF can reduce the risk of thromboembolic stroke through initiation of anticoagulation. Rapid response to AF can be identified and managed before inappropriate shocks are delivered. Regarding when to begin remote monitoring, in the setting of ambulatory (same-day discharge) device implant, the author has found that having the patient perform a remote transmission the day following implant to be highly useful.

Challenges to remote monitoring include maintaining a connection between the device and the transceiver. Although with a dedicated proprietary unit, this mostly involves keeping the latter connected to a power source, with newer devices that communicate with a cell phone application, this requires leaving the application open at all times. Note that although remote monitoring is highly recommended in the guidelines, an annual in-person visit is also recommended to assure proper operation of automated features and to make adjustments to the device as needed.

Personally, the author has always found it interesting that follow-up scheduling is primarily based on astrological events (each time the earth travels around the sun, ie, 1 year, the patient will be seen back for evaluation. With that in mind, current recommendations are as follows:

Class-1(A): Remote CIED monitoring with 1 annual in-person evaluation is recommended over a calendar-based schedule of in-person evaluations alone.

Class 1(A): All patients with CIEDs should be offered remote monitoring as part of standard follow-up.

Class 1(E): Before starting remote follow-up, patients should be educated as to the nature of remote monitoring, their responsibilities, expectations, potential benefits, and limitations.

Class 1(A): Remote monitoring should be performed to monitor lead function and battery status.

Class 1(E): Remote monitoring should be performed for devices that have been recalled or are on alert for early detection of actionable events.

Class 1(B-R): Remote monitoring of ICDs should be performed to reduce the incidence of inappropriate shocks (mostly from lead malfunction and atrial arrhythmias such as AF with rapid ventricular response and supraventricular tachycardias [SVTs]).

Class 1(A): Remote monitoring should be performed to monitor for early detection and quantification of AF.

Class 2A(C): Remote monitoring should be initiated within 2 weeks of CIED implantation.

Specifically for Implantable Loop Recorders

Class 1(E): All patients should be enrolled in remote monitoring given the availability of data on a daily basis.

Additional recommendations for staff expertise and data management are also made in this document. These recommendations include the following:

Class 1(E): Staff involved in interpreting transmissions and managing patients should be qualified in the same manner as those doing in-office evaluations (ie, they should be International Board of Heart Rhythm Examiners [IBHRE] certified or equivalent). Note: this recommendation was made before the availability of the specific remote monitoring certification offered by IBHRE as of 2021.

Class 1(E): Policies, procedures, roles, and responsibilities should be codified as written policy, especially as to the timeliness of evaluation and notification of findings.

REMOTE PROGRAMMING

Currently, there are no remote programming guidelines; as for other than ILRs, no remote programming is possible. The latest generation of ILRs now allows for remote programming of several parameters, eliminating the need for patients to present in person for changes to sensitivity, heart rates, and pause lengths. Because ILRs do not have any therapeutic functions, this has been deemed as "safe." However, it will not be long (in the author's opinion) until remote programming is available for pacemakers and ICDs. Once that function becomes available, guidelines will be needed and are likely to appear in the literature.

HEART FAILURE MONITORING

Although heart failure monitoring had been available through measurement of chest wall impedance for many years, the low specificity of the initial algorithm made for many false positive events. The newer-generation algorithms as well as the combination of multiple measured parameters have allowed for significant strides in sensitivity and specificity. In most cases, the heart failure parameters are a "bonus" feature incorporated into a CIED, although newer-generation ILRs may be able to be used for this purpose as well. There does appear to be broad acceptance for payment (at least in the United States) for monthly monitoring of devices for heart failure. Note that there is a dedicated pulmonary artery (PA) pressure monitor, the CardioMEMS device from Abbott Medical. This device is interrogated once every 24 hours to determine the PA pressure. However, reimbursement for management of patients with this device is inconsistent and depends on the payer. The detection of arrhythmias, such as AF, runs of VT, SVT, and frequent PVCs, that contribute to the presence or worsening of heart failure, can be detected early by monitoring. Current guidelines[4,6] suggest the following:

Class 1: Frequent interrogation or remote monitoring of stored arrhythmia episodes in device-implanted heart failure patients should be performed in order to diagnose AF and allow its early management.

Class 1: Interval use of ECG and arrhythmia-directed monitoring for development of AF-induced cardiomyopathy and risk assessment over time should be part of standard follow-up for patients with AF.

Class 2b(C): Remote monitoring may be used to manage heart failure.

QT INTERVAL PROLONGATION, QT VARIABILITY, AND ST SEGMENT CHANGES

Although ambulatory monitoring can be used to detect these changes on the ECG, there are no guidelines for performing monitoring for the sole reason of evaluation for this purpose.[2] ST changes can be detected to diagnose ischemia owing to atherosclerotic disease as well as Prinzmetal angina.

Although a standard 12-lead ECG is typically used for measuring the QT interval and for changes as a result of drug treatment, ambulatory ECG and MCOT can also be used to assess efficacy of drug treatment and its potential adverse effects, such as bradycardia and proarrhythmia. These same modalities may be used for evaluation of increased QT variability/dispersion, which are considered markers of electrical instability and therefore related to higher risk of sudden cardiac death.

BRADYCARDIA

Most symptomatic bradycardia and conduction disorders are intermittent and may necessitate a longer term of heart rhythm monitoring. Correlation of symptoms and rhythm is very desirable. For symptoms occurring daily, a 24- or 48-hour continuous ambulatory ECG (Holter monitor) is often adequate and cost-effective. For those with more intermittent symptoms, longer-term monitoring is best. The current guideline[3] for detecting bradycardia is as follows:

Class 1(B-NR): In the evaluation of patients with documented or suspected bradycardia or conduction disorders, cardiac rhythm monitoring is useful to establish correlation between heart rate or conduction abnormalities with symptoms, with the specific type of cardiac monitor chosen based on the frequency and nature of symptoms, as well as patient preferences.[3]

VENTRICULAR TACHYCARDIA

Different types of monitoring may be used to evaluate a patient for the presence, frequency, and complexity of VT. Monitoring may also be used to assess the efficacy of therapy, or to correlate symptoms with the rhythm. The type and duration of monitoring will depend on the frequency of the suspected arrhythmia, and the intent of the monitoring. The 2017 guideline for VT suggests the following[9]:

Class 1(B-NR): Ambulatory ECG monitoring is useful to evaluate whether symptoms, including palpitations, presyncope, or syncope, are caused by ventricular arrhythmias post-myocardial infarction patients.

Class 2a: In patients with sporadic symptoms (including syncope) suspected to be related to VA, implanted cardiac monitors can be useful. Implanted cardiac monitors provide continuous rhythm monitoring and stored recordings of electrograms based on patient activation or preset parameters, allowing a prolonged monitoring period of a few years.

NONISCHEMIC DILATED CARDIOMYOPATHY

There are many causes of nonischemic dilated cardiomyopathy, including infiltrative, PVC induced, pacemaker induced, autoimmune, metabolic, toxic, inherited, and tachycardia mediated. Although ambulatory ECG monitoring may be considered for risk stratification relative to life-threatening ventricular arrhythmias, the prognostic value of this type of surveillance is low, relatively nonpredictive, and remains controversial. There are no guidelines that recommend routine monitoring of this population.[2]

ARRHYTHMOGENIC RIGHT VENTRICULAR CARDIOMYOPATHY/DYSPLASIA (ARVC/D)

Patients with arrhythmogenic right ventricular cardiomyopathy (ARVC) have a high risk of heart failure and sudden cardiac arrest/death (SCA). In addition, because this is often a genetically transmitted disorder, first-degree relatives of the patient may be at risk as well.[2] Frequent PVCs and nonsustained VT are risk factors for SCA. Initial evaluation of all patients suspected for ARVD/C should include 24-hour ambulatory ECG monitoring. Current guidelines are as follows:

Class 1(B-NR): Patients and first-degree relatives should be screened by 24-hour ambulatory

ECG every 1 to 3 years starting at age 10 to 12 for excessive (>1000) PVCs, which is a major risk factor, or greater than 500 PVCs (minor risk factor).[10]

Class 2: In patients with confirmed ARVC, regular Holter monitoring and imaging for assessment of ventricular function may be useful.[6]

HYPERTROPHIC OBSTRUCTIVE CARDIOMYOPATHY

Although in hypertrophic obstructive cardiomyopathy the hallmark of the disease is the hypertrophy of the septum, the left ventricular outflow tract gradient and the presence of ventricular arrhythmias on ambulatory monitoring (Holter) are also important risk factors for the patient.[6] In addition, the presence of AF may result in worsening of symptoms, such as congestive heart failure.[2] Syncope and palpitations may be the result of AF, PVCs, VT, SVT, outflow tract obstruction, or even neurally mediated events. American College of Cardiology Foundation/AHA guidelines initially published in 2011 recommended 24-hour ambulatory ECG monitoring; however, the 2014 ESC guidelines recommend 48 hours. The most recent guideline[6] does not specify a duration.

Class 1: Ambulatory ECG evidence of nonsustained VT provides prognostic information and is recommended.

CHAGAS DISEASE

Nonsustained VT is part of the Rassi mortality risk score (3 points).[6] This score should be obtained by a 24-hour ambulatory ECG monitor. Determining the Rassi score is a class 1 recommendation, so it follows that obtaining this type of study would follow as a class 1 recommendation.

WOLFF-PARKINSON-WHITE

The use of ambulatory ECG monitoring is potentially useful in patients with Wolff-Parkinson-White for evaluation of accessory pathway conduction properties. If, during ambulatory recording, intermittent preexcitation or rate-related loss of preexcitation is present, this is suggestive of a lower-risk pathway owing to the latter having a longer refractory period. Thus, the guideline for monitoring is as follows[6]:

Class 2: Noninvasive screening with exercise testing, drug testing, and ambulatory ECG monitoring may be considered for risk stratification in asymptomatic preexcitation patients without high-risk occupations or those who are not competitive athletes.

LONG QT SYNDROME

Long QT syndrome is a group of hereditary channelopathies characterized by QT prolongation. The resultant ventricular arrhythmias may result in syncope, cardiac arrest, or sudden death. There are some variants that are noted for prolongation of QT interval and/or inappropriate QT adaptation to heart rate. In addition, arrhythmias are frequently preceded by R-R variation (ie, long-short cycles). However, at this time, there are no recommendations in the guidelines for any type of heart rhythm monitoring to diagnose, establish treatment, or help in the decision to implant an ICD. The presence of syncope in the absence of a long QT diagnosis should be evaluated as described above. The 12-lead ECG remains the gold standard for diagnosis of long QT syndrome.[2,6] However, there are guidelines for monitoring patients with an established diagnosis of an inherited arrhythmia for ambulatory ECG monitoring:

Class 1: Patients with certain inherited arrhythmia syndromes are at higher risk for AF and benefit from symptom-driven and periodic surveillance.

Class 1: Evaluation should include noninvasive symptom-driven surveillance for patients at risk for AF and periodic noninvasive surveillance for asymptomatic patients.

SHORT QT

Short QT syndrome is a channelopathy diagnosed in patients with QTc $\leq$ 340 milliseconds. These patients have a predisposition to AF and SCA without the presence of structural heart disease. Patients may be asymptomatic or present with SCA as the initial presentation. Although ambulatory ECG monitoring may be helpful to determine the cause of syncope and palpitations, there is no other role in diagnosis or guiding therapy.[2,6] However, refer to the guidelines for long QT syndrome above.

BRUGADA

Brugada syndrome is an inherited sodium channelopathy causing a predisposition to VT/fibrillation and death. As the ECG of patients with Brugada syndrome is highly variable and can fluctuate over time, it has been suggested that ambulatory ECG monitoring might provide diagnostic and/or prognostic information for affected patients. It has even been noted that the characteristic ST changes are more notable in the afternoon hours. The idea of using 12-lead or "high" V1 and V2 electrode locations to diagnose Brugada syndrome has also been put forward, although not accepted into any guideline at this time. Screening for AF, ST-T wave alternans, spontaneous left bundle branch block, and PVCs has also been suggested. In patients with undiagnosed syncope, longer-term ambulatory ECG recording (with or without special lead positions) or ILR placement can be considered.[2,6] Guidelines otherwise follow those of inherited disorders, as described for long QT syndrome.

CATECHOLAMINERGIC POLYMORPHIC VENTRICULAR TACHYCARDIA

Although uncommon, catecholaminergic polymorphic ventricular tachycardia is a lethal inherited channelopathy. Exercise or emotion-driven increases in sympathetic tone and catecholamine levels result in palpitations, syncope, and possibly SCA because of ventricular arrhythmias. Ambulatory ECG monitoring is useful to assess the presence of ventricular tachyarrhythmias during activities and emotional stress. An exercise stress test is used to evaluate the relationship of ventricular arrhythmia with increased catecholamines. Ventricular ectopy develops and is proportional to frequency and complexity with higher heart rates. Atrial arrhythmias may also occur with stress. Ambulatory ECG was recommended in the past to evaluate the efficacy of drug therapy; however, this has not made it into the current guideline, which follows that as for long QT syndrome. One reason is that the presence of asymptomatic PVCs on monitoring does not imply an unfavorable prognosis.[2,6]

EARLY REPOLARIZATION SYNDROME

Early repolarization syndrome is characterized by J-point elevation in the inferior and/or lateral leads. It has been associated with idiopathic ventricular fibrillation (VF) and SCA. Earlier guidelines suggested that ambulatory ECG monitoring may contribute to documentation of this disorder; however, it has been found that the 12-lead ECG finds most affected patients. Although an increase in J-point elevation amplitude preceding ventricular arrhythmias has been reported in with electrical storm, there are no recommendations for monitoring other than those for inherited arrhythmias, as noted above.[2,6]

IDIOPATHIC VENTRICULAR FIBRILLATION

Idiopathic VF is defined as a resuscitated cardiac arrest with ECG documentation of VF, in subjects in whom cardiac, respiratory, metabolic, and toxicologic causes have been excluded. Although it has been suggested that evaluation of survivors include ambulatory ECG as well as other diagnostic tests, the current guidelines do not include ambulatory or other rhythm monitoring for further diagnosis, as placement of an ICD is usually the next step before discharge from the hospital. There may be a role for ambulatory ECG monitoring of first-degree relatives of idiopathic VF victims.[2]

DIALYSIS AND CHRONIC KIDNEY DISEASE

End-stage renal disease (ESRD) is characterized by mortality of up to 20% per year, with a cardiovascular death rate 100 times higher than the general population. Sudden cardiac death is the most common cause of death in these patients. Data on the rate of asymptomatic ventricular cardiac arrhythmias based on ambulatory ECG recording in patients with ESRD have been conflicting. Although there is a higher incidence of AF in patients on hemodialysis, there are no guidelines specific to this population regarding heart rhythm monitoring.[2,6]

NEUROLOGIC AND MUSCULAR DISEASES

This group of patients is characterized by a disturbance in the autonomic nervous system that can be studied by ambulatory ECG. Analysis of ambulatory ECG looking for a reduction in heart rate variability may be particularly helpful. These patients are prone to both bradyarrhythmias and tachyarrhythmias. Faster heart rates have been documented before neurologically mediated seizures owing to epilepsy.

Myotonic dystrophy a genetic condition that is associated with block at various sites in the heart's conduction system. It is also associated with AF and VT. Thus, sudden death may be due to atrioventricular (AV) block or ventricular arrhythmias. Although ambulatory ECG monitoring may be used to detect arrhythmias and to guide device choice, there are insufficient data to provide a guideline for its use.[2,6]

SLEEP APNEA

Sleep apnea syndrome (sleep-disordered breathing) is common and affects 2% to 4% of the population. Arrhythmias and conduction system disorders have been clearly associated with this disorder. The diagnosis is made by polysomnography, which includes ECG monitoring. This type of testing is not always readily available, and it has been suggested that use of ambulatory ECG monitoring might at least partially assist in making the diagnosis. Some commercial ambulatory monitoring units provide apnea analysis using breathing-related changes in sinus rhythm, and changes in R-wave amplitude modified by respiratory movement of the chest wall as a surrogate for respiratory rate/depth. However, no guideline for the use of ambulatory ECG for this purpose exists yet. Most often, sinus pauses or the presence of Mobitz-1 AV block during early morning hours (typically associated with sleeping) presents the suggestion that there is a diagnosis of sleep apnea syndrome.[2]

POSTVENTRICULAR TACHYCARDIA AND PREMATURE VENTRICULAR COMPLEX ABLATION

Following ablation of ventricular arrhythmias or PVCs, surveillance for efficacy and recurrence of the arrhythmia or PVC is recommended. Surveillance should be performed immediately after and then after a short recovery period, especially in patients without an ICD or other device that can identify and quantify the rhythm.[2] Interestingly, the most recent joint society document on VT ablation[11] has no particular guideline on postablation monitoring. An earlier HRS/EHRA consensus statement from 2009[12] recommended ambulatory ECG monitoring for 4 weeks around the follow-up interval. This ambulatory ECG monitoring should include symptom-triggered recordings and weekly transmissions for asymptomatic episodes. Also recommended is 24- to 72-hour Holter monitoring or 30-day autotriggered event monitoring or ambulatory ECG during a minimum follow-up of 6 to 12 months (regular monitoring of arrhythmia during this period of time).

POSTATRIAL FIBRILLATION ABLATION

Patient symptoms alone tend to both overestimate and underestimate the presence of AF, both before and after ablation. Therefore, reliance on symptoms alone is insufficient to characterize the success and durability of an ablation. If a patient does not have an implanted device, extended ambulatory ECG monitoring helps to identify the presence, frequency, and duration of postablation AF. Complete absence of AF is a particularly good prognostic indicator. Recurrences in the "blanking period" (typically about 3 months postablation) may require medical therapy and/or cardioversion.

HRS guidelines suggest a 24-hour ambulatory ECG monitor at 1 year, and event recording regularly and at the time of symptoms. It is recommended that monitoring continue periodically from 3 to 12 months following ablation of paroxysmal AF. For persistent AF, this document suggests 24-hour ambulatory ECG monitoring at each 6 months

after ablation, and event-driven ECG monitoring as needed. As noted above, in some cases ILR implant may be used to monitor long term for AF burden after ablation. Reimbursement may be problematic and depend on the payer for this intervention.[2]

POSTPHARMACOLOGIC TREATMENT ASSESSMENT

Management of AF patients using a rate control strategy is common. Utilization of pharmacologic agents to reduce symptoms and to minimize the change of a tachycardia-associated cardiomyopathy is key to the management of this arrhythmia. The basic guidelines regarding rate control for AF are noted in later discussion; however, monitoring may also be used to evaluate for rhythm control, with the goal of a reduction in AF burden or elimination of the arrhythmia. Use of ambulatory monitoring may also provide insight regarding proarrhythmic effects of new pharmacologic therapy (new or increased ventricular ectopy, prolongation of the QT or QRS, atrial flutter with 1:1 conduction, postconversion pauses, and so forth).[2]

Class 2(A): Ambulatory ECG monitoring is useful to achieve a target heart rate at rest averaging no higher than 80 bpm.

Class 2(B): Ambulatory ECG monitoring is useful to achieve an average heart rate of 100 to 110 bpm during the monitoring period.

EVALUATION OF CARDIAC IMPLANTABLE ELECTRONIC DEVICE FUNCTION AND ARRHYTHMIAS

Although modern CIEDs have complex diagnostics and are capable of storing large amounts of data (including electrograms), they are not always able to identify the cause of a patient's symptoms, nor are they capable of detecting certain malfunctions (eg, undersensing, failure to capture, pacemaker-mediated tachycardias, upper rate behavior). Ambulatory ECG monitoring can provide a diagnosis and correlate device function/malfunction with patient symptoms. Recommendations for monitoring patients with CIEDs are based on the same general principles as discussed above and are based on the severity, frequency, and duration of the patient's symptoms.[2]

POSTURAL ORTHOSTATIC TACHYCARDIA SYNDROME/VASOVAGAL SYNCOPE/ INAPPROPRIATE SINUS TACHYCARDIA

Patients who are being evaluated for these disorders of the autonomic nervous system frequently present significant challenges. Ambulatory

ATHLETES AND PRECOMPETITION SCREENING

Athletes present a challenge for monitoring, given that symptoms often occur during the type of activity that requires significant physical exertion. Some sports, such as swimming, present significant challenges for all external monitors available. Rarely, symptoms suggestive for arrhythmia can be a sign of impending SCA, or may indicate a serious but treatable rhythm disturbance. A basic ECG and other noninvasive tests, such as treadmill stress and echocardiogram, are initially performed to evaluate for stress-induced arrhythmias and the presence of an underlying structural abnormality. If the symptom or arrhythmia is not reproducible, ambulatory ECG is useful. As always, the type of monitoring depends on symptom frequency, severity, duration, and inciting factors at the time of the symptoms. As noted, some types of athletics may preclude certain types of monitoring options.[2] **Box 1** lists the low- and high-risk features for syncope, and these should be considered when pursuing a diagnosis.

SUMMARY

Guidelines exist for monitoring to diagnose and manage patients with many different conditions. Although there have been recent updates to the guidelines, the constantly evolving and advancing nature of the technologies creates a gap at times between the newest monitors, the indications for their use, and reimbursement by the payers. The key element to the choice of the modality of monitoring remains matching the correct technology to the type, severity, frequency, and duration of the patient's symptoms.

CLINICS CARE POINTS

monitoring may prove helpful in some cases. For those with infrequent syncope, possibly owing to vasovagal syncope, longer-term monitoring may be useful. Longer-term monitoring would include the use of an ILR. Other syndromes that have more frequent symptoms can be evaluated with shorter-term monitoring. The guideline for inappropriate sinus tachycardia is as follows[13]:

Class 2b: A 24-hour Holter monitoring may be useful (diagnostic average heart rate >90 bpm over 24 hours, resting heart rate of >100 bpm).

- Match the type of monitoring to the frequency, duration, and severity of the clinical symptoms.
- Implantable monitors should be used only when longer-term monitoring is required, or when a patient is unable or unwilling to comply with wearable monitors.
- Matching symptoms to recorded events is critical to make a diagnosis or exclude heart rhythms as the cause of the symptoms.

DISCLOSURE

Medical Consultant: Medtronic, Philips Image Guided Therapy. Research Support: Boston Scientific. Honoraria: Abbott Medical, Convatec.

REFERENCES

1. Shen WK, Sheldon RS, Benditt DG, et al. 2017 ACC/AHA/HRS guideline for the evaluation and management of patients with syncope. Heart Rhythm 2017; 14:e155–217.

2. Steinberg JS, Varma NJ, Cygankiewicz I, et al. 2017 ISHNE-HRS expert consensus statement on ambulatory ECG and external cardiac monitoring/telemetry. Heart Rhythm 2017;14:e55–96. International Society for Holter and Noninvasive Electrocardiology.

3. Kusumoto FM, Schoenfeld MH, Barrett C, et al. 2018 ACC/AHA/HRS guideline on the evaluation and management of patients with bradycardia and cardiac conduction delay. Heart Rhythm 2019;16: e128–226.

4. Slotwiner D, Varma N, Akar J, et al. HRS Expert Consensus Statement on remote interrogation and monitoring for cardiovascular implantable electronic devices. Heart Rhythm 2015;12:e69–100.

5. Gorenek B, Bax J, Boriani G, et al. Device-detected subclinical atrial tachyarrhythmias: definition, implications and management—an European Heart Rhythm Association (EHRA) consensus document, endorsed by Heart Rhythm Society (HRS), Asia Pacific Heart Rhythm Society (APHRS) and Sociedad Latinoamericana de Estimulación Cardíaca y Electrofisiologíia (SOLEACE). Europace 2017;19: 1556–78.

6. Nielsen JC, Yenn-Jiang L, de Oliveira Figueiredo MJ, et al. European Heart Rhythm Association (EHRA)/Heart Rhythm Society (HRS)/Asia Pacific Heart Rhythm Society (APHRS)/Latin American Heart Rhythm Society (LAHRS) expert consensus on risk assessment in cardiac arrhythmias: use the right tool for the right outcome, in the right population. Heart Rhythm 2020;17(9):e269–316.

7. January CT, Wann LS, Calkins H, et al. 2019 AHA/ACC/HRS focused update of the 2014 AHA/ACC/HRS guideline for the management of patients with atrial fibrillation. Heart Rhythm 2019;16(8): e66–93.

8. Mairesse GH, Moran P, Van Gelder IC, et al. Screening for atrial fibrillation: a European Heart Rhythm Association (EHRA) consensus document endorsed by the Heart Rhythm Society (HRS), Asia Pacific Heart Rhythm Society (APHRS), and Sociedad Latinoamericana de Estimulacióon Cardíaca y Electrofisiología (SOLAECE). Europace 2017;19: 1589–623.

9. Al-Khatib S, Stevenson WG, Ackerman MJ, et al. 2017 AHA/ACC/HRS guideline for management of patients with ventricular arrhythmias and the prevention of sudden cardiac death. Heart Rhythm 2018; 15:e73–189.

10. Tobin JA, McKenna WJ, Abrams DJ, et al. 2019 HRS expert consensus statement on evaluation, risk stratification, and management of arrhythmogenic cardiomyopathy. Heart Rhythm 2019;16(11): e301–72.

11. Cronin EM, Bogun FM, Peichl P, et al. 2019 HRS/EHRA/APHRS/LAHRS expert consensus statement on catheter ablation of ventricular arrhythmias. Heart Rhythm 2020;17(1).

12. Aliot EM, Stevenson WG, Almendral-Garrote JM. EHRA/HRS expert consensus on catheter ablation of ventricular arrhythmias. Europace 2009;11: 771–817.

13. Sheldon RS, Grubb BP, Olshansky B, et al. 2015 Heart Rhythm Society expert consensus statement on the diagnosis and treatment of postural tachycardia syndrome, inappropriate sinus tachycardia, and vasovagal syncope. Heart Rhythm 2015;12(6): e41–63.

Data Management and Integration with Electronic Health Record Systems

Gerald A. Serwer, MD

KEYWORDS

- Structured reporting • Electronic health record • Cardiac implantable electronic device
- Cardiac device remote monitoring • IDCO profile

KEY POINTS

- Need for smooth and reproducible data flow from device to the electronic health record that is vendor agnostic.
- Need for standardized data nomenclature.
- Need for standardized data flow and interchange format.
- Need for standardized reporting format.
- Need for creating a report tailored to the needs of the intended recipient (electrophysiologist, general cardiologist, primary care provider, and patient).

A long anticipated benefit of the development of the electronic health record (EHR) system has been the automatic data acquisition, transfer, and integration among various systems ranging from those that collect patient data to the final repository, the EHR. In general, parts of this have been realized, but much has not. More importantly, issues have arisen that were initially unsuspected that have plagued the further development of this needed functionality. In this work, the author outlines the current state of data management, transfer, and integration and highlights remaining problems that exist as they pertain to the cardiac implantable electronic device (CIED). The ideal state would be that information is created by the CIED and then transferred to multiple systems with no manual data entry or data manipulation to positively affect patient care while minimizing data error. Unfortunately, this is not yet the situation. For this discussion, the author uses information generated by CIEDs to illustrate data transfer and utilization with the problems that exist.

CIED remote monitoring is able to retrieve information from a patient's device without requiring the patient to come to the clinic and electronically forward it to the responsible physician. Such systems now can interrogate the patient's device automatically without any interaction with the patient. This information is then sent to a unique central receiving system for each vendor for processing and transmission to the responsible physician. Unfortunately, every vendor of such devices has chosen to do it differently, and thus, a single system capable of receiving information from all vendors has been difficult to achieve. In some works,[1] there is a distinction made between remote interrogation and remote monitoring. Remote interrogation implies retrieval of information from the device specific to its functionality, including battery longevity. Remote monitoring denotes information retrieved from the device specific to intercurrent patient events with criteria preprogrammed into the device. For the purpose of this article, no distinction is made between these two, and the term remote monitoring refers to both types of information. The author discusses specific elements necessary to ensure unambiguous data acquisition and transmission of

University of Michigan, UM Congenital Heart Center, Michigan Medicine, 11-715Z Mott, SPC 4204, 1540 East Hospital Drive, Ann Arbor, MI 48109-4204, USA
E-mail address: gserwer@umich.edu

Card Electrophysiol Clin 13 (2021) 473–481
https://doi.org/10.1016/j.ccep.2021.05.001
1877-9182/21/© 2021 Elsevier Inc. All rights reserved.

information in a vendor-neutral manner together with elements considered necessary but not yet necessarily in existence. This discussion is followed by a schema of data flow from the originating CIED to the EHR and patient portal.

REQUIRED ELEMENTS FOR SMOOTH DATA TRANSFER

In order to attain the smooth flow of information, data requirements must exist that include the following:

- Unambiguous patient identification
- Unambiguous device identification
- Standardized semantic and syntactic data nomenclature
- Common data transfer methodology/interchange format
- Structured reporting of the information relevant to the consuming audience

Patient and Device Identification

A unique patient identifier (UPI) has long been discussed dating back to the late 1990s. However, it raises issues relevant to potential patient privacy and required action at a national level to account for patient relocation. Privacy concerns have led to its lack of funding for many years, but, it is hoped, the UPI will be addressed in the immediate future, as funding legislation is now being considered.[2]

A universal device identifier (UDI) has been implemented by the federal government that begins to address the question of unique identification of implantable hardware and linkage of all implanted components to form a unique system for a given patient. All implanted devices and hardware are required to have a UDI that can easily be read using a standard bar code. This use of the standard bar code eliminates the need for manual data entry of device identifying information and greatly decreases the change of data entry error. Linkage of a given patient and a given system allows for patient and device tracking that is essential for the clinician to be able to deal with device recalls and the potential problems that they can cause.

Common Data Syntax

One of the major recent accomplishments is the creation of a structured data set.[3] This allows for a specific semantic description of the data elements together with a syntactical structure that can then be transformed into a human readable report, as is discussed later (**Fig. 1**), and provides an IEEE-compliant framework within which

additional elements can be added over time. This allows for unequivocal entry of data elements whose meaning does not change from vendor to vendor. As cardiac devices evolve, additional elements can be added, and existing elements can be altered or deleted as needed. Some elements are now designated as required or mandatory that must be sent, if present, for data compliance versus optional, where its inclusion in the data stream is left to the discretion of the vendor. Clinician and societal input is crucial in assigning either mandatory or optional status to each element. Work by the Heart Rhythm Society on adding newer data elements and assignment of mandatory/optional status will soon be available. Currently, there are approximately 180 data elements.

Message Transmission

The data elements are then placed in a standard HL7 message for transmittal to either a third-party Cardiac Data System or the EHR. Currently, the message format used is HL7 V2.6. However, this allows for only one-way information flow. Work is ongoing to use bidirectional data flow protocols, for example, HL7's FHIR, that would allow additional data from the third-party vendor or EHR to be added to enhance the reporting capabilities of the system. An example is the exchange of scheduling information for subsequent sessions between the EHR and Cardiovascular Information System (CVIS) vendors.

Structured Reporting and Presentation

As the CIED in most instances has only minimal patient-identifying information, patient identification must be added to the data set. This can come from a registry table that associates a given UDI to the proper patient. This can be maintained by either a CVIS or the EHR. Such a table requires a mechanism for maintaining accurate associations when a new CIED is placed in a patient. Such an association must be addressed for new implantation. The incorporation of a Universal Patient Identifier within the CIED would obviate this problem.

Once the message is received by the reporting entity, for example, EHR, it must be translated from the IEEE nomenclature to a more readable form and placed in a structured report format so that all reports irrespective of the device vendor present the same information in the same manner to increase clinician usability. The major feature is to present the key information needed by the consumer, be it a general care physician, electrophysiologist, or the patient. Often several report formats are needed to address the different

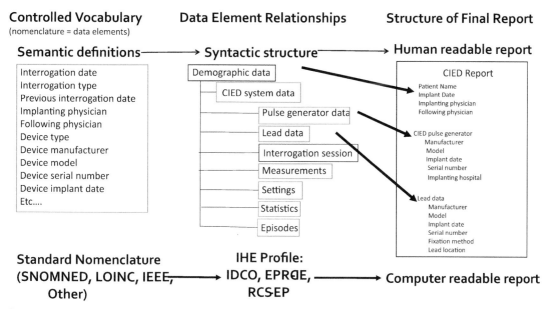

Controlled Vocabulary
(nomenclature = data elements)

Data Element Relationships

Structure of Final Report

Fig. 1. Controlled vocabulary flow from the semantic definition of the data elements to the syntactical structure of all elements and then translated into a human readable report. (*From* Slotwiner D. Electronic health records and cardiac implantable electronic devices: new paradigms and efficiencies. Journal of Interventional Cardiac Electrophysiology. 2016;47(1):29-35. https://doi.org/10.1007/s10840-016-0170-1; with permission.)

consumers. This is a potential weakness, as the translation from IEEE nomenclature to more readable text is dependent on the EHR or third-party vendor, and no deviation from the prescribed data element definition can be allowed. Ideally, this is performed by a large group of stakeholders with the same translation used by all vendors while still allowing for vendor-to-vendor variation.

PROCESS FLOW SUMMARY
Implantable Device Cardiac Observation Profile

In 2011, the Patient Care Domain of the Integrating the Healthcare Environment (IHE) published a method (or profile) to transfer information from a CIED remote interrogation to an EHR encompassing many of the above requirements.[4] This was entitled "Implantable Device–Cardiac–Observation" or IDCO profile. It stipulated a method to unambiguously transmit such data. This profile stipulated a methodology to address many of the above requirements.

For remote monitoring of cardiac devices, the data flow proposed by the IDCO profile is summarized in **Fig. 2**. The implanted device (CIED) is interrogated by the vendor-specific device remotely or in the device clinic with all collected data transferred to the interrogating device in a vendor-specific proprietary manner. For remote monitoring, it is then sent to the vendor-specific Web site in a proprietary format. For in-clinic interrogation, it is

sent to a third-party CVIS in varying formats where it is then reviewed and validated by the clinic personnel and translated from proprietary to IEEE nomenclature observing the data syntax and semantics specified in the IEEE data standard. It is next reviewed by the responsible clinician and forwarded via a defined HL7 message to the EHR. In some cases, the EHR can also function as the CVIS reviewing system, having received the data directly from the vendor Web site. In the EHR, it is used to create a standardized report for consumption by the clinician and patient. Each EHR deals with this in a different manner. If bidirectional data flow is available, the data now in the third-party CVIS can be combined with EHR data for a more informed and complete report.

Another key issue is the point along the path at which the clinician assigned to the report reviews and approves the data, completing the report. This can be either be within the CVIS before transmission to the EHR or within the EHR after the data are received if the EHR is also functioning as a CVIS. Assignment of the physician responsible for report completion must be performed in a reproducible manner. There is a data element within the IEEE nomenclature for transmittal of the responsible physician identification allowing it to be added at any point. The EHR has the capability to further forward the information in the IEEE format to implant registries or national quality improvement registries.

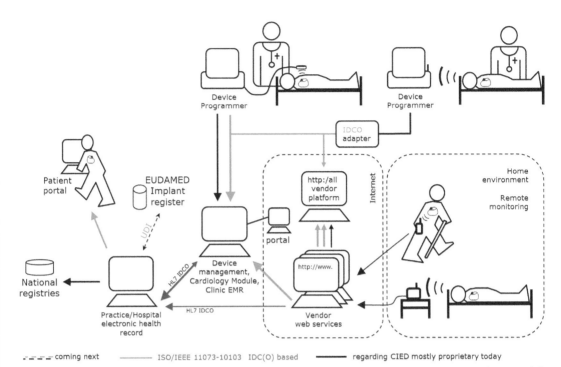

Fig. 2. The IDCO profile schematic diagram of data flow from either an in-clinic interrogation at the top of the diagram or a remote interrogation (*right*) to the vendor-specific Web site for interpretation or downloading to the third-party data manager (CVIS or clinic electronic medical record [EMR]) where it is processed and finalized before being sent to the EHR. The data may or may not be translated into IDCO format by the device programmer before transmittal to the clinic EMR. Once in the EHR, the finished report can be accessed directly by the clinician or via a patient portal. Exportation of the data to a national registry or implant register is possible. EUDAMED, European Union Medical Device Registry. (*From* Slotwiner D, Abraham R, Al-Khatib S et al. HRS White Paper on interoperability of data from cardiac implantable electronic devices (CIEDs). Heart Rhythm. 2019;16(9):e107-e127. https://doi.org/10.1016/j.hrthm.2019.05.002; with permission.)

To this point, all data have been in either numeric or textual form. Electrogram waveforms (EGMs) are sent by most CIEDs and are of interest to the clinician. The IDCO profile data stream does have the ability to include such waveforms in the data stream as an encapsulated and Base64 binary encoded PDF file. This requires clinician review of the available waveforms to pick which ones to attach to the data stream. Of note is that the attached PDF file must contain the particulars related to its significance (eg, date and circumstances of acquisition) needed to place the EGM in the proper context.

Data Security and Patient Responsibility

Finally, data security is not addressed directly in the IDCO profile but is clearly needed if the data stream uses a public network. Also, it becomes potentially a privacy issue if data are stored on systems remote to the local health system environment. The European Union via the General Data Protection Regulation enacted in 2016 places legal responsibility for documenting data transmission and place of storage upon the "data controllers."[5] Such controllers may be device manufacturers and/or health systems, and the responsibilities of each must be specified. This regulation provides a common legal framework that stipulates how patient personal information is collected, managed, and stored and a structure of accountability for data security. It stipulates that, although remote monitoring can be offered to all patients with such devices, specific consent must be obtained. This included the right of the patient to withdraw consent with their data purged from the affected databases or moved to a different provider system receiving their data "in a structured, commonly used and machine-readable format."[5] This portability relies on the principles described previously, again emphasizing the importance of all systems that interact with such information using a common data syntax as well as transport protocol. It has been proposed that patients should be informed how their monitored information will be secured and used. Currently, in the United States, there is as yet no such national regulation. Nevertheless, data transparency does guarantee patients access to their medical information, including these CIED data pieces.

Some centers do obtain signed patient permission for patient enrollment, and others do not. Even among centers acquiring written authorization, there is great variability as to the content of the permission form. Usually, this form is composed of the following:

- Patient acknowledgment that the device will send information via the device vendor to the responsible center
- Goals of remote monitoring and the patient benefits
- What remote monitoring does and does not provide
- Medical personnel involved
- Clinic responsibilities to the patient
- Patient responsibilities
- Consequences of patient noncompliance
- Charges to the patient/insurance

Ideally, such a consent should be obtained at the time consent for the implant procedure is obtained before the procedure. The consent form should be uniform across centers so that if the patient changes health care providers, a new form is not needed. Having a standardized consent form accepted by all health care organizations would greatly simplify this consent process and make patient transfer from one system to another much easier.

DATA INTEGRATION INTO THE ELECTRONIC HEALTH RECORD

Once the information arrives in the EHR in a standardized form, several issues still need to be addressed within the EHR.

First, the information to be presented in the report must be decided on. This is guided by the intended audience for this information. Information intended for use by electrophysiologists is often more extensive than information required by the patient via a patient portal. If this is not addressed appropriately, either too much information is provided and the intended message may be overwhelming to the patient, or too little information is provided and the important message about their device function is not conveyed. Work by Daley and colleagues[6,7] defines the data thought to be important to the patient. This can be addressed by having the same data populate multiple reports, allowing the provider and patient to select the appropriate one to meet their needs.

Second, the terminology data provided by the IDCO profile, while unambiguous, are often unclear to the casual reader. Some elements require little explanation. By example, "Comments" is quite understandable. However, others are not clear; **Fig. 3** provides examples. In addition, one must decide how to provide for data that are not present in a given report. An example would be to simply say that a data element is "not present" or to leave the data field blank. A third option would be to remove the data label as well as the

Reference ID Prepend MDC_IDC_	Display name	Definition
SESS_DTM	Date time of interrogation session	Date and time of the in-clinic or remote interrogation session
SESS_TYPE	Type interrogation session	The type of device interrogation that generated the current data set
SESS_REPROGRAMMED	Reprogrammed during session	Indication of whether the device was reprogrammed during the session
SESS_DTM_PREVIOUS	Date time previous interrogation session	Date and time of a previous in-clinic or remote interrogation
SESS_REPROGRAMMED_PREVIOUS	Re-programmed during previous session	Indication of whether the device was reprogrammed along with the previous interrogation
SESS_CLINICIAN_NAME	Clinician name	Name of the clinician that is responsible for the examination
SESS_CLINICIAN_CONTACT_INFORMATION	Clinician contact information	Contact information for the responsible clinician

Fig. 3. Sample data element nomenclature from the IDCO schema with the corresponding display name, and definition. Must prepend the string "MDC_IDC_" to each term in column 1 for it to be fully IEEE compatible. IDC, implantable device cardiac; MDC, medical device communication.

Patient Name:	Doe, John	IEEE 11073-10101
Date of Birth:	Jan 1 , 1940	IEEE 11073-10101
Gender:	Male	IEEE 11073-10101

Interrogation Date, Type	Oct 25, 2007 10:00 AM, Remote
Previous Interrogation Date, Type, Program:	Sep 25, 2007 10:00 AM, In-Clinic, (Reprogrammed)
Clinician Name, Clinic	Dr. Anderson, Main Heart Center New Jersey
Clinician Contact	Phone: +1 12 345 6789, e-mail follow-up-physician@clinic.org

Device Demographics

Device Type:	CRT-D
Device Manufacturer:	Manufacturer Name
Device Model:	Device Model Name
Device serial Number:	5867463524
Device Implant Date:	May 1, 2005
Device Implanter, Facility:	Dr. Miller, Main Heart Center New York
Device Implanter Contact:	Phone: +1 12 345 6789

Lead Demographics

	Lead 1	Lead 2	Lead 3	....
Lead Location Chamber:	RA	RV	LV	
Lead Location Detail:	Appendage	Apex	Free wall	
Lead Implant Date:	05/01/2005	05/01/2005	05/01/2005	
Lead Manufacturer:	Vendor Name	Vendor Name	Vendor Name	
Lead Model:	SuperSense	SuperSense	SuperSense	
Lead Serial Number:	1234657812	1234567813	1234567814	
Lead Polarity Type:	Unipolar	Bipolar	Bipolar	
Lead Connection Status:	Connected	Connected	Connected	
Lead Special Function:	Pressure Sensor			

STATUS/ MEASUREMENTS

Battery:	08/25/2007	Capacitor	(most resent charging)
Battery Status:	MOS	Charge Date:	June 1, 2006 10:00 AM
Battery Voltage:	6.3 V	Charge Time:	8.1 s
Battery Impedance:	2500 ohms	Charge Energy:	36 J
Battery Remaining:	75% 4 y 11 mo	Charge type:	Reformation

RRT (ERI) Trigger:	Battery voltage <5.7 V / Cap. Charge time >12 s

Fig. 4. A possible structured report proposed using the IDCO nomenclature. (*From* Slotwiner D, Abraham R, Al-Khatib S et al. HRS White Paper on interoperability of data from cardiac implantable electronic devices (CIEDs). Heart Rhythm. 2019;16(9):e107-e127. https://doi.org/10.1016/j.hrthm.2019.05.002; with permission)

space for the intended data element. Nevertheless, whatever method is chosen, this must be done in a uniform and consistent manner.

Third, the structure of the report for different classes of devices must be decided on. It is imperative that all patients with a similar device, for example, pacemaker versus implantable cardioverter defibrillator, versus implanted loop recorder, have the same report structure, as this makes quickly scanning the report much easier and less prone to overlook critical data elements. If the structure of the report is known to the reader, obtaining specific information needed is much quicker and less fraught with potential error. Not all institutions will choose to use the same report structure, but this structure must be consistent throughout a given institution. This is not unique to this type of data, but a consistent reporting structure is highly recommended throughout all medical reporting. The structured report or reports ideally are the same in all health care systems, but variation will occur. **Fig. 4** provides in part an

example of a structured report provided in the IDCO profile. An example of a partial report used in the author's local institution is shown in **Fig. 5**. The report should consist of several segments designed to convey information in the order needed. Each section has both mandatory and optional information with the minimal set of information acceptable.

The first section identifies the patient as well as the report date and type of device present followed by a summary of the findings and the report date and time. The remainder provides details that may or may not be needed in all cases. The next section identifies the hardware present as well as electrode locations. This is followed by measurement information providing battery status, electrode functionality (impedance and threshold), and device events, such as percent of pacing in each chamber, high rate events, and therapies delivered (if applicable).

This is followed by a more detailed description of episodes together with the outcome of the

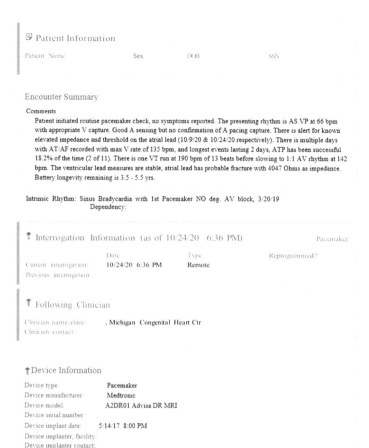

Fig. 5. A portion of the author's local structured report as seen by the clinician in the EHR.

therapy delivered. Finally, device-programmed settings are provided. The rationale is to provide the most used information early in the report followed by less often needed and unchanging information toward the end.

WORK FLOW ISSUES

The first issue is the point at which the report is reviewed and finalized by the responsible clinician. There are at least 3 possible sites at which this can occur. The first is within the device vendor Web site if it allows entry of a comment or summary statement. This generally is the least customizable of the available options but does not require investment in additional software and training. It produces a report that is the hardest to electronically transmit except as a fixed file (eg, PDF file).

The next option is a third-party or middleware vendor. The CVIS receives the information from the manufacturer site or sites and presents it in a common manner independent of the device manufacturer. It is often customizable to meet individual needs, but this functionality can be limited. The clinician reviews the information and enters a summary statement before sending it to the EHR. In this setting, the EHR acts only as a data receiver. This assures that only reviewed and verified information is available to the other patient providers and the patients themselves. Nevertheless, the time delay in getting the information to the EHR can be the longest, as it requires an extra step.

Finally, the EHR itself can act as both the data receiver from the device manufacturer Web site and the point at which the clinician reviews and confirms the information. This eliminates transmittal of the finished report to the EHR as it is completed within the EHR but does potentially allow viewing of nonverified information depending on the EHR configuration.

Option 1 is the simplest to configure but provides the least flexibility. Options 2 and 3 are in some ways similar but are quite variable from both a middleware vendor and an EHR vendor perspective.

The next area to consider is how to efficiently address device alerts. Alerts are of 2 types.

Most are reports of events and therapies delivered, appropriate or inappropriate. The second type is reports of system (device or electrode) malfunction. It is estimated that alerts of all types can occur in up to 55% of patients during a single year.[8] Depending on the number of patients followed, this can be a large number that must be evaluated and addressed, requiring significant personnel time. Some alerts may require no intervention, but all do require evaluation.

SUMMARY

Movement of information from an implantable device (CIED) to an EHR can be a complex and multi-step process consisting of transmission to a vendor-specific site, then to a middleware vendor for clinician review, and finally to the EHR. It requires a unique patient and device identifier through the use of the universal patient identifier and the UDI. This ensures unambiguous transmission of the information from its origination in the device to its ultimate home in the EHR. This methodology also allows transmission to multiple endpoints. Use of a common and agreed on terminology by all vendors decreases the work needed to provide an accurate interface between the source and the receiver and data uniformity across device vendors. Data transmission requires secure transmission techniques and data encryption to protect patient privacy. Once the information arrives in the EHR, it must be converted to an agreed on terminology and easily understandable form. Ideally, there should be several forms of this report appropriate for the information consumer, for example, the patient, the primary care physician, the cardiologist, and the electrophysiology specialist.

Although remote monitoring has been the standard of care since publication of the first Heart Rhythm Society consensus document in 2015,[9] it is not universally used. Whether this is because of physician or patient reluctance is unclear. Certainly, there are legal barriers, appropriately aimed at protecting patient privacy and patient rights to control their medical information, but, it is hoped, this will not diminish the advantages that this technology provides particularly in this period of uncertainty and the desire to decrease visits to medical facilities without a decrease in the quality of care delivered. Remote monitoring data transmission serves as a model for other forms of discrete medical data transmission from source to EHR minimizing transcription errors and improving patient care.

CLINICS CARE POINTS

- Use of a standardized data nomenclature reduces report ambiguity and enables comparison between data from different device manufacturers and eliminates possible misinterpretation of the data.
- Use of a structured report format allows for more quickly finding the required information in the report irrespective of the device manufacturer.
- Structured reporting allows for easily creating a report tailored to the needs of different report consumers, for example, electrophysiologist, general cardiologist, primary care provider, and patient.
- Standardized data nomenclature and structured reporting allow for easy transferability of device information should the patient change care providers.

DISCLOSURE

None.

REFERENCES

1. Slotwiner DJ, Abraham RL, Al-Khatib SM, et al. HRS White Paper on interoperability of data from cardiac implantable electronic devices (CIEDs). Heart Rhythm 2019;16(9):e107–27.
2. Luthi S, Cohen JK. House votes to overturn ban on national patient identifier. 2019. Available at: http://www.modernhealthcare.com/politics-policy/house-votes-overturn-ban-national-patient-identifier.
3. ISO/IEEE 11073-10103:2014. Health informatics — point-of-care medical device communication — Part 10103: nomenclature — implantable device, cardiac. 2014. Available at: https://www.iso.org/standard/63904.html.
4. Kraus A, Schultz T, Steblav N, et al. Implantable device - cardiac - observation (IDCO) profile. 2011. Available at: https://wiki.ihe.net/index.php/PCD_Implantable_Device_Cardiac_Observation.
5. European Union. Regulation (EU) 2017/745 of the European Parliament and of the Council of 5 April 2017 on medical devices, amending directive 2001/83/EC, regulation (EC) No 178/2002 and regulation (EC) No 1223/2009 and repealing council directives 90/385/EEC and 93/42/EEC. Available at: http://eur-lex.

europa.eu/legal-content/EN/TXT/?uri=uriserv:OJ.L_.
2017.117.01.0001.01.ENG&toc=OJ:L:2017:117:TOC.

6. Daley C, Toscos T, Mirro M. Data integration and inter-operability for patient-centered remote monitoring of cardiovascular implantable electronic devices. Bioengineering 2019;6:25.

7. Daley CN, Chen EM, Roebuck AE, et al. Providing patients with implantable cardiac device data through a personal health record: a qualitative study. Appl Clin Inform 2017;8:1106.

8. O'Shea CJ, Middeldorp ME, Hendriks JM, et al. Remote monitoring alert burden. An analysis of transmission in > 26,000 patients. J Am Coll Cardiol 2020. https://doi.org/10.1016/j.jacep.2020.08.029.

9. Slotwiner D, Varma N, Akar JG, et al. HRS expert consensus statement on remote interrogation and monitoring for cardiovascular implantable electronic devices. Heart Rhythm 2015;12:e69.

Organizational Models for Cardiac Implantable Electronic Device Remote Monitoring
Current and Future Directions

Carly Daley, MS[a,b,*], Tammy Toscos, PhD[a,b], Tina Allmandinger, BSN, RN[c], Ryan Ahmed, MS[a], Shauna Wagner, BSN, RN[a], Michael Mirro, MD, FACC, FHRS, FAHA[a,b,d]

KEYWORDS

- Arrhythmia • Electrophysiology • Cardiovascular implantable electronic device
- Remote monitoring • Organizational models • Workflow

KEY POINTS

- The use of remote monitoring (RM) of cardiac implantable electronic devices (CIEDs) has been shown to improve clinical and economic outcomes.
- The explosion of data from RM transmissions will require the use of advanced technologies (machine learning/artificial intelligence) to relieve the cognitive burden on the CIED team and ensure quality care.
- Standardization of reports across implantable CIED vendors will improve clinic performance and minimize errors (professional societies, such as the Heart Rhythm Society, should provide guidance, credentialing opportunities, and other support toward standardization).
- Development of reporting of CIED data output that is tailored to individuals will improve patient engagement and support patient–provider shared decision making about disease management.

INTRODUCTION

The ability of remote monitoring (RM) for cardiac implantable electronic devices (CIEDs) to improve both clinical and economic outcomes is now clear.[1] Devices are growing in complexity and sophistication, and the number of patients with CIEDs who require ongoing management is increasing.[2] Despite the evidence for efficacy and need, RM adoption among electrophysiology (EP) practices over the past decade has not been consistent.[3,4] One of the major barriers to adoption is the lack of guidance for how to manage RM data and patient follow-up. Currently, the structure and organization of RM clinics are heterogeneous.[5] Focusing on the optimization of clinic models is a priority for improving RM adoption and efficiency,[6] a need that became more urgent during the COVID-19 pandemic, when the Heart Rhythm

[a] Health Services and Informatics Research Department, Parkview Mirro Center for Research and Innovation, 10622 Parkview Plaza Dr., Fort Wayne, IN 46845, USA; [b] Department of BioHealth Informatics, IUPUI School of Informatics and Computing, 535 W. Michigan St., Indianapolis, IN 46202, USA; [c] Arrhythmia Diagnostic Center, Parkview Physicians Group, 11108 Parkview Circle, Fort Wayne, IN 46845, USA; [d] Department of Medicine, Indiana University School of Medicine, 340 West 10th St., Indianapolis, IN 46202, USA
* Corresponding author.
E-mail address: carly.daley@parkview.com

Card Electrophysiol Clin 13 (2021) 483–497
https://doi.org/10.1016/j.ccep.2021.04.008
1877-9182/21/© 2021 Elsevier Inc. All rights reserved.

Society (HRS) urged clinicians to conduct remote CIED interrogation as much as possible.[7]

This review builds on the work describing RM in EP practice by Mittal and colleagues[8] and Ricci and Morichelli,[6] with the goal of providing key considerations to clinicians and health care administrators who are creating or strengthening a RM clinic model.

The purpose of this review is to

1. Provide an overview of organizational models for RM clinics
2. Describe the benefits and challenges of existing RM clinic models
3. Present a case report on an RM clinic that is implementing a new workflow
4. Provide considerations for the management of RM data and recommendations for the organization, staffing, and structure of an RM clinic

ORGANIZATIONAL MODELS FOR REMOTE MONITORING MANAGEMENT

The technical capabilities for RM and complexity of devices have surged in the past several years. RM of CIEDs began with transtelephonic monitoring of pacemakers in the 1970s and since has evolved into more sophisticated interrogation systems allowing for increased RM in lieu of in-office checks. Remote access to CIED data has an impact on patient care, improves outcomes, and decreases mortality,[8] and RM is now part of the guidelines for CIED standard of care.[9]

Organizational models for the workflow are needed in order to effectively implement the guidelines for RM follow-up.[10] Studies on the impact of RM have had different outcomes partially due to factors related to the variations in set-up and workflow.[11] In practice, the implementation of RM is heterogeneous between clinics due to the variation in the manufacture of devices and associated Web sites, lack of standardized workflow and organizational model, and lack of reimbursement models.[12,13]

Several European studies evaluated organizational workflows or models over the past decade (**Table 1**). The studies implemented different types of models and overall demonstrated that having a specialized team to monitor RM transmissions streamlined workflow. According to Ricci and Morichelli, 3 main models for RM workflow are (1) the external centralized call centers model, which involves a specialty team that has the capability to monitor thousands of patients on a 24 hours per day/7 days per week basis, with EPs on call; (2) the hub and spoke model, where 1 center monitors and screens RM data for several smaller satellite

clinics; and (3) the primary nursing model, where a nursing office manages the home device delivery, patient training, monitoring, and screening of data, and reporting critical events to the physician.[6]

Among the various models, the primary nursing model has been increasingly observed over the past several years.[4,20] This may be because nurses can dedicate time to reviewing transmissions while also maintaining contact with patients and knowledge of patient history, thus reducing the amount of time required for physicians to review the data.

Importantly, the organizational model should be specialized for CIED RM monitoring and involve staff trained in the management of CIEDs, or a CIED team.[21] Zanotto and colleagues[21] recommend that the CIED team include 3 or more CIED-certified allied health professionals (nurses and/or technicians), and Lucà and colleagues[22] suggest that specialized CIED staff should include a referring nurse and supervising physician. The concept of the CIED team, with trained allied health professionals working closely with a physician, maps to the primary nursing model. **Table 2** provides more implementation details on the roles and responsibilities of allied health professionals and physicians as part of a specialized CIED team.

Similar to other countries, RM has not been utilized in all arrhythmia centers in Italy despite known benefits.[4] According to a recent survey study, however, the rate of RM use in Italy increased from 86% (in 2012) to 98.2% (in 2017) among 57 centers (out of 183 that participated) that completed surveys at both timepoints.[4] The following changes were observed over time at these centers, reflecting the trend toward the primary nursing model:

- Increased involvement of cardiac physiologists (technicians) and decreased involvement of number of personnel from the device manufacturing companies
- Increase in number of nurses and technicians (and decrease in number of physicians) conducting primary review of RM reports
- Increase in the number of transmissions shared with physicians only if critical events occurred and decrease in the total number of transmissions shared with physicians

Additionally, an informed consent process was used at both time points; however, there was a significant increase in the use of the informed consent form made available by the Italian Association of Arrhythmology and Cardiac Pacing. Both surveys showed that only clinically significant events that required a follow-up action were reported to

Table 1
Studies evaluating or assessing remote monitoring organizational models and workflows

Author, year	Patients	Setting	Study Design	Model Type	Description	Outcome Measures	Key Findings
Müller et al,[14] 2013	55 ICD or CRT-D patients (1 device vendor)	Germany, 10 clinical sites and 1 telemedical service center	Prospective, multicenter, nonrandomized, observational study	Hub and spoke model	• Trained professional staff • Patients' medical history and medication were known • APs defined by study protocol	• Patient and physician satisfaction • Alert filtering	• Mean follow-up of 402 d ±200 d • Total 3831 AP identified; 682 sent to 10 sites; 46 resulted in action taken by the clinic.
Vogtmann et al,[15] 2013	121 PM and ICD patients (1 device vendor)	Germany, 9 clinical sites and 1 monitoring center	Prospective, nonrandomized, multicenter, observational study	Hub and spoke model	• Monday–Friday, 8:00 AM–4:00 PM • Two trained TNs and 2 physicians • TNs classified data as red, yellow, or green	• Feasibility and safety of the workflow • Time effort • Consequences of forwarded messages • Value of forwarded messages	• Mean follow-up of 445 d ±133 d for ICD and 340 d ±160 d for PM • 1649 event notifications per 100 patients/y • TN 30 min/d and physician 1.1 min/d per 100 patients monitored • 131.8 messages (including 148.8 events) were sent to clinics.

(continued on next page)

Table 1
(continued)

Author, year	Patients	Setting	Study Design	Model Type	Description	Outcome Measures	Key Findings
							• Clinics took action on 37.3% of all messages. • 72.3% of messages rated as valuable
Ricci et al,[16] 2014	1650 PM and ICD patients (1 device vendor)	Italy, 75 sites	Multicenter observational study	Primary nursing model	• Each patient assigned to an RN and RP • RN filters HM data. Reviews within 2 working days upon HM alert. Critical reports sent to RP. Followed written protocol • Involved initial patient training	• Time per outpatient clinic personnel for patient follow up activities • Outpatient clinic workload • Resource consumption	• Median follow-up 18 (10–31) months • 3364 HM sessions performed • 723 actionable events • 43.3 RNs and 10.2 RPs min/mo/100 patients • 48% of patients were called; 58% of calls were to restore transmissions and 38% for unscheduled in-hospital visits.
Guédon-Moreau et al,[17] 2015	562 ICD patients (4 device vendors)	France, single site	Prospective, single-center, observational study	Primary nursing model	• Nurses and cardiologists working together • Defined roles for nurses • Decision trees	• Time spent managing transmissions and alerts	• Decrease in clinical and technical alerts by 21% (1.53 alerts/patient/y) • Decreased time spent on alerts by half • Decreased variability in time spent by nurses

Study	Setting	Patients	Study design	Organizational model	Model description	Objectives	Results
Dario et al,[18] 2016	Italy, 6 cardiology departments	1871 PM and ICD patients (5 device vendors)	Multicenter, multivendor, controlled, observational, prospective study	Primary nursing model	EP nurse/technician: • Reviews data daily through vendor Web portals • Sends data to physician when there is an event • Contacts patient as necessary for instructions	• Effectiveness and efficiency of RM for PMs and ICD compared with in-clinic • Timeliness of detection of acute episodes recorded by the device, workload, and direct costs	• Nurses spent 48% of time inserting data into the EHR and communication with patients. • Contact with patients was regarding connection problems for 26% of PM and 14.3% of ICD • The numbers of false alerts were 42.2% (PM) and 27.1% (ICD)
Giannola et al,[19] 2019	One hospital site in Italy	153 PM and ICD patients (1 device vendor)	Single-center observational study	External RM center/primary nursing hybrid	• One trained nurse and 1 supporting physician • Clinical history available • Daily check to Web site • All transmissions reviewed within 1 working day • Transmission color code (red-amber-green) classification in predefined protocol • High-priority events (red) were sent by phone and email to the hospital	• Feasibility of outsourcing remote triage to an external center • Time to review all transmissions	• Mean 8.4 (SD 1.1) mo of follow-up • 613 transmissions per 100 patient-years • Red transmissions required urgent care in 60% of cases; 92% of amber events managed remotely • Time from transmission to review reduced from 11 (4–25) d to <24 h (0–1 d) • During standard follow-up, 21% of transmissions not reviewed after 1 mo; with ERMC all transmissions reviewed within 2 working days

Abbreviations: AP, actionable parameter; ERMC, external remote monitoring center; HM, home monitoring; ICD, implantable cardioverter defibrillator; PM, pacemaker; RN, reference nurse; RP, responsible physician; TN, telemonitoring nurse.

Table 2
Defined roles and responsibilities for staff in a specialized cardiac implantable electronic device team

Zanotto et al,[21] 2020	CIED certified nurses and/or technicians • Collaborate with CIED companies (technical support for remote consulting) • Manage ambulatory and in-hospital patients • Maintain relationship and communication with patients and their care network (approximately 700–1000 patients per nurse/technician) • Filter alerts before consulting with physicians (who are available daily for alerts) • Execute different workflows depending on cardiac conditions (atrial fibrillation, heart failure, and ventricular arrhythmias)	Physician • Be available for daily review of alerts and consult with nurses and technicians
Lucà et al,[22] 2019	Referring nurse • Provide patient education • Enter patient data into Web site • Review alerts within a predefined time • Screen data to identify false negatives and verify programming of alerts • Call patient when there is a transmission interruption • Coordinate with physician for review of critical cases. • Establish written algorithm to standardize process of alerts • Follow-up with patients in office after implant and yearly in office thereafter	Supervising physician • Obtain informed consent • Supervise organization • Evaluates critical events • Contact general physician and specialists • Coordinate with referring nurse for review and to evaluate critical events

patients. As has been reported elsewhere, lack of reimbursement was a consistent barrier to RM.[4,12]

CONSIDERATIONS FOR REMOTE MONITORING MANAGEMENT
Data Standardization and Interoperability

According to Mittal and colleagues,[8] 3 primary goals of the EP practice for the management of CIED data are to (1) have efficient access to CIED data, (2) extract clinically valuable information, and (3) present information clearly in the electronic health record (EHR). These 3 goals require standardization and interoperability of the data. Currently, there are disparate types of data from different manufacturers, each with its own Web site, proprietary nomenclature, and communication protocols.[23] For example, battery status and percent biventricular pacing both are presented in different ways across device manufacturers.

In order to standardize the data in common interfaces, third parties must normalize the data so that they can be presented in a way that is consistent, easy to read, and makes sense to the end user. One solution for standardization and interoperability is the implantable device cardiac observation (IDCO) profile, which leverages existing standards, such as Health Level Seven. Beginning in 2006, organizations, including Integrating the Healthcare Enterprise, Institute of Electrical and Electronics Engineers, and HRS, and industry, collaborated on the development the profile. The IDCO profile has afforded clinics a more streamlined process leading to time savings, error reductions, and increases in efficiency and patient safety.[24]

Reducing Data Overload and Alert Burden

RM systems can capture a large amount of data from CIEDs. The data are not always actionable, however. A study following patients with devices from 4 different vendors over a period of 1 year found that only 42% of events were actionable.[25] The relatively low rate of actionable events and frequency of alerts can lead to alert fatigue. For example, device manufacturers each provide a unique set of parameters for alerts, leading to an increased volume of alerts to clinics that manage a population with various device types. Furthermore, certain CIEDs have a poor signal to noise ratio (ie, implantable loop recorders), which also contributes to an increased volume of alerts stemming from false-positive results generated by under or oversensing.[26] Even when alerts are programmed by physicians, there still are many transmissions that do not generate actionable alerts, and only a small fraction of alerts require immediate attention.[27]

A recent study found only 40.2% of incoming transmissions were actionable (yellow or red). Thus, 60% of all transmissions were nonactionable (green); 38% were yellow alerts, and 2% were red alerts.[27] This ratio could create a bottleneck effect in the clinic, when attending to the incoming transmissions and trying to ensure that actionable alerts are addressed as soon as possible (**Fig. 1**). Because the management of alerts takes place during office hours, delays can result from processing time to catch up on transmissions that occurred over the weekend.

Standardization of alert acuity is challenging due to the lack of consistent alert parameters and definitions as well as context.[27] For example, the severity of an AF episode may be different for a nonanticoagulated patient who does not have a history of AF compared with someone who is on anticoagulant and does have a history of AF. Tailoring of alerts individually is more realistic and effective than standardizing different episodes for alerts[27] and should begin immediately post-implant.[28]

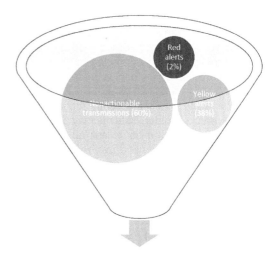

Processing and follow-up

Fig. 1. Depiction of the bottleneck effect that occurs with the number of transmissions incoming to the clinic. (*Data based on* O'Shea CJ, Middeldorp ME, Hendriks JM, et al. Remote Monitoring Alert Burden: An Analysis of Transmission in >26,000 Patients. *JACC: Clinical Electrophysiology.* 2020.)

Engaging Patients in Remote Monitoring

Over time, RM technology has evolved away from wand-based monitoring to landline, and now wireless options, making it easier for patients and clinicians. Although RM reduces the resources required for in-office visits,[29] there are new workflow challenges created by RM, such as following up with patients for missed RM transmissions. Engaging patients in a way that encourages the recommended use of RM is an essential part of patient care.

In order to engage patients in RM for optimal clinical outcomes and patient satisfaction, it is important to understand the advantages and disadvantages of RM from the patients' perspectives. For example, RM makes care more accessible and reduces travel time, and patients may appreciate being monitored by clinicians and experience improved health outcomes.[30] On the other hand, RM can lead to decreased interaction and contact with patients,[31,32] apprehension about being monitored,[33] and loss of unstructured time to ask general questions about underlying cardiac disorders.

Although general satisfaction with RM may be consistent[34] regardless of factors, such as age,[35] certain populations still may desire the opportunity to have in-office checks. For example, Timmermans and colleagues[32] found that 43% of the 300 participants (median age 66) preferred in-clinic visits; the median age of this subgroup was 67 (interquartile range 60–74). Geriatric patients who are at risk of effects of isolation and loneliness[36] may find benefit in coming to the clinic to see their health care providers in person. Additionally, Kelly and colleagues[5] found that satisfaction with clinic visits was consistently higher for patients 70 years and older. Patients may prefer in-office visits due to the ability to ask questions and likely would prefer to not have remote checks exclusively.[5] Thus, it is important to consider a hybrid model of virtual and in-office visits as well as investigate how to optimize the sense of connection with RM.

Older adults also may be more likely to have misconceptions about RM compared with younger adult patients.[35,37] Although this has not been shown to have an impact on adherence, prior work shows the value of education, information, and support to help close gaps in understanding among patients. Toward this goal, 5 categories of communication can be considered by those who are designing patient engagement interventions: diagnostic work (eg, finding out patients' symptoms in order to interpret device data), inclusion work (eg, helping the patients use their home monitor and resolve disconnection), coordination work (eg, scheduling), education work (eg, explaining how the CIED works), and comfort work (eg, reassurance about being monitored).[38]

Addressing Disparities in Remote Monitoring Follow-up

There is legitimate concern that an increased focus on RM may widen the gap in health care access that already exists among minoritized and underinsured/uninsured groups unless efforts are made to engage people appropriately and equitably. There is a known disparity in follow-up visits post-CIED implant, evidenced in a study of 38,055 Medicare beneficiaries in the United States. Despite an overall increase in the number of follow-up visits post implant between 2005 and 2009, initial follow-up visits were higher among white patients than Black patients and patients of other races, and were more likely for patients in the age range of 65 to 79 than patients of ages ≥ 80.[39]

Social conditions also play a role in uptake of RM. For example, in a large study with 269,471 patients in the United States, completing at least 4 years of college and having a landline or cell phone in the home were positive predictors of RM, whereas living below the poverty line, lack of health insurance, unemployment, not in the work force, lower median income, and living in an urban neighborhood were predictors of less RM use.[40] Providing patients with cell phone adapters free of charge has been shown to improve adherence to RM regardless of race and among people who live in urban areas.[41] Rosenfeld and colleagues[42] studied compliance among a real-world population undergoing RM and found that age, geographic location, and clinic size were clinically relevant factors in RM compliance. Older patients (>80) had a significantly lower rate of noncompliance as compared to both groups of middle-aged patients (age 41-80) and younger patients (40 years or younger).[42] Thus, the diversity of social needs, as well as perceptions of and preferences for RM, across the patient panel in a clinic has relevance for engagement, uptake and adherence to RM.

Impact of Missed Transmission and Disconnected Monitors on Workflow

Another important part of RM patient care is following-up with patients who have issues with interrupted transmissions or disconnected monitors.[19] Disconnected monitors are a concern to nurses because of increased workload and because patients may be under a false assumption that they are being monitored when in fact their monitor is disconnected.[43] There are implications for patient outcomes, because transmission interruptions could potentially lead to missed alerts of clinically significant events.[44] The implications on workload in the clinic include increased phone calls to inform patients and troubleshoot disconnected monitors.[15,16] Many instances of disconnected monitors and missed transmissions can be resolved by the patient plugging in their monitor or ensuring they are within range for the monitor to detect their device,[15] suggesting that improved methods of education and supportive interventions could reduce the amount of time and work spent calling patients and troubleshooting.

Data Privacy and Security

Concerns about responsibility of RM data and medicolegal issues present a barrier to adopting RM.[4,45] There is concern regarding medical liability for not including certain RM alerts and allowing too much time to review and respond to transmission data.[22] An implication for clinic workflow is that patients should be informed of the caveat that RM is not for emergency situations and that remote programming is not performed through RM.[22] Additionally, there should be measures for ensuring compliance with Health Insurance Portability and Accountability Act and General Data Protection Regulation within the clinic, such as documentation of informed consent processes. Some of the concerns about receiving and monitoring RM data for patients can be alleviated through utilizing the IDCO profile. As 1 clinic reported, utilization of the IDCO profile helps mitigate security concerns by connecting patient data from the manufacturer Web site to the EHR, reducing errors through seamless integration.[24]

FUTURE OF REMOTE MONITORING MANAGEMENT
Use of Middleware to Manage the Data

With the different device vendors and management systems for RM, the pathway to universalization of RM has been complex.[46] The disparate sources and formats of data intensifies the work burden.[28] In order to help organize data across various sources, middleware platforms, were established to help clinics pull data from different vendors while reducing the need for hardware, such as floppy disks.[47] The industry of middleware platforms, also described as third-party vendors or universal RM platforms, to help organize RM data has expanded over the past decade with companies providing advanced functionalities that facilitate workflow.[48] Third-party middleware companies have different features and functionalities. Some of these features include

1. Integrating data from CIED vendors into EHRs
2. Utilizing and supporting the IDCO profile
3. Providing RM interpretations as a service
4. Customizing reports for clinics (such as a heart failure report)
5. Facilitating scheduling
6. Managing for missed transmissions
7. Providing software as a service model
8. Providing revenue management as a service model
9. Utilizing cloud-based data storage

One of the challenges that third-party middleware companies face is that they have to deal with the specifications of the device manufacturers and the format and availability of data as well as the specifications of the EHR platforms that they interface with to make data available to clinicians (**Fig. 2**).

Each implantable device vendor organizes and presents the data in different formats, and that typically requires integrating data from 3 to 4 manufacturers per clinic. The middleware assists by integrating the different sources and presenting information in a single interface.

One of the roles of professional societies (that lead the development of practice guidelines (e.g. HRS)) will be to create standardization of reporting, to enhance semantic interoperability. Using the same lexicon and vocabulary is an important foundational element for error reduction, data accessibility, enhancing data quality and communication.

Sharing Data with Patients

As technology improves, patients may have more access to data and use specific apps to check the manufacturers' Web sites and communicate with their care team.[22] Device manufacturers have patient-facing applications; however, the amount of actual data shared with patients related to their health monitoring is limited. Research shows that patients have an interest in receiving their data[49] and that it is feasible to deliver data to patients without having an impact on clinic workload.[50] Care must be taken, however, to understand how patients want to receive their data (how much and what information is needed to help them interpret the data).[51–53] There is an ethical responsibility to ensure that patients understand their data and respond appropriately, with an accurate level of interpretation and without causing unwarranted concern.[53,54] Providing patients access to their CIED data is aligned with the legal rights individuals have to access their own information[55] and is part of the paradigm shift in RM.[56]

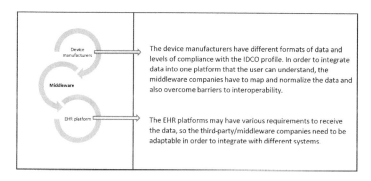

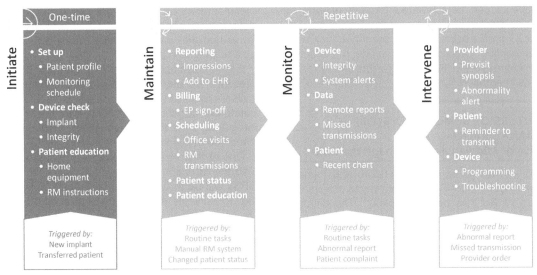

Fig. 3. Workflow in the ADC in terms of the tasks involved.

Patients may have questions about their data that may lead to extra phone calls to the clinic. They may be able, however, to resolve more issues on their own (such as disconnected monitors). Having access to alert data prior to receiving a call from the clinic could create anxiety; alternatively, it may help the patients receive the medical advice given to them during the phone call, because they will have had more time to process the information. Patients who are engaged in their health and have the cognitive, emotional, and physical capacities to monitor and learn from their data may benefit the most from having access to their data. To avoid widening the disparities among people who receive the most benefit from

their device, care must be taken to address issues in technology, perceptions of RM, and personal health, life goals, and values of patients as well as cognitive and physical requirements, to make sure that the solutions are tailored to meet individual needs.

REMOTE MONITORING CLINIC CASE EXAMPLE

The following case example is from the perspective of the clinic supervisor. The Arrhythmia Diagnostic Center (ADC), located in a large not-for profit hospital system in the Midwest, has applied the primary nurse model to deliver RM care. The ADC has a dedicated CIED management team

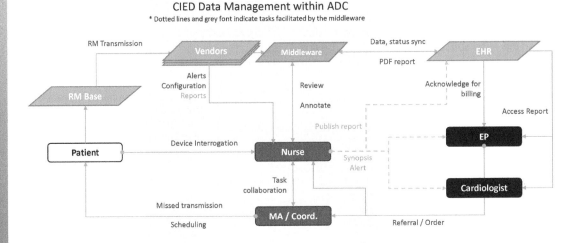

Fig. 4. Workflow in the ADC following the path of the CIED data. Coord, coordinator.

Table 3
Key considerations for remote monitoring management based on the major points of the review

Considerations for EP clinics	Related to RM clinic organization	• Optimize overall effort, resources, and patient care with a dedicated staff (such as CIED team) with defined roles and responsibilities • Include a physician medical director (implanting EP) and a nurse administrative leader managing clinic operation, aligning with the primary nursing model • Provide routine education for the CIED team on evolving CIED technologies and review of complex clinical cases seen in the clinic, and include participation in a certification process and/or documentation of a minimum level of competency • Leverage systems (such as middleware) to help with tasks such as scheduling and patient notification of upcoming transmissions for wand-based remote devices • Implement a hybrid model of remote, virtual, and in-office visits to accommodate patients' needs
	Related to data management	• Focus support and efforts toward the adoption of the IDCO profile for downstream effects on improved ease and workflow • Allocate time and resources to the activity of tailoring of alerts for patients to improve signal to noise ratio of alerts • Integrate a middleware system designed to interface directly with the hospital EHR in order to help with efficiency; consider a support team consisting of both clinical and information technology professionals in the early days of implementation
	Related to clinic workflow	• Account for follow-up with patients that is aimed toward obtaining their health information and knowledge to help with data interpretation • Make efforts to increase patient engagement and enhance interactions to make up for reduction of in-person interactions • Identify ways to provide patients with education and support throughout the course of monitoring to help them feel reassured as well as give timely information (eg, helping patients understand how the monitor works to facilitate troubleshooting if there is a disconnection) • Provide patients with assistance, such as cell phone adapters to improve adherence to RM

Considerations for vendors and developers		• Recognize that while emerging technology allows for more data capture and sophisticated algorithms, there needs to be end-user design, interpretation, and use cases built into the output
		• Include key stakeholders in the design and development of technologies of RM such as
		  ○ Clinic staff because they understand the needs and pain points from both clinical and administrative perspectives
		  ○ Patients and informal caregivers, who can inform design of technologies for patient-facing interfaces bidirectional communication

Considerations for policymakers		• Facilitate progress of standardization and interoperability, through a solution such as universal adoption of the IDCO profile, and certification process • Provide clarity and transparency for data privacy, security, patient education, and consent as well as guidance on how clinics can measure adherence to the regulations

with one nurse supervisor, six nurses, a clinic coordinator, and a medical assistant (MA). On a given day, two nurses are dedicated to RM while three nurses see patients in the clinic. Sometimes the supervisor sees patients as well. The MA answers the phone, sends out letters to patients, and is not involved in direct patient care. There is an ADC coordinator, who schedules patients for in office visits, assists with triaging phone calls, and manages the clerical side of the department. The tasks in the ADC are depicted in **Fig. 3**.

Affordances of a New Middleware System

The ADC is undergoing a transition to a new middleware system designed to directly interface with the hospital EHR in order to help with efficiency. Middleware allows centralized management of data from multiple vendors, reducing the amount of time it takes for managing data, scheduling, ensuring billing intervals are correct. Thus, the software reduces the administrative tasks for the clinic staff so they can focus more time and effort on reviewing clinical information and providing individualized patient care.

The number of remote transmissions that staff are able to process into full reports for clinicians and physicians to review is expected to double with the help of the middleware to manage the data. The system can improve efficiency by pulling impressions from the transmissions, allowing nurses to review for accuracy rather than having to pull the impressions manually. The nurses edit text in the impressions box as needed. Additionally, the system was built at this site to interface directly with the EHR, eliminating the need to scan in reports and allowing clinicians outside the ADC to see data (discrete and portable document formats (PDFs)) from remote transmissions immediately after processing, and only 1 report must be signed by the EP per billing cycle (per quarter). This also allows for easier tracking of accurate billing cycles. The ADC bills for 4 remote cycles and sees the patient yearly in the clinic, allowing for complete tracking and documentation of remote follow-ups. **Fig. 4** shows the workflow of the RM data in the ADC, highlighting the role of the middleware system.

Challenges to Middleware Implementation

The transition to middleware has some challenges. For example, after a month of implementation, the system was backlogged partially due to reconciling historical and current data in 1 system. The ADC supervisor anticipated that it will take some time for the clinic to reach their efficiency goals. The middleware company created an interface with the EHR for this health system, exploring new territory for both the middleware company and the ADC, and requiring robust testing and troubleshooting. Thus, it may be helpful to have a support team consisting of both clinical and information technology professionals working closely with the ADC clinic in the early days of implementation.

KEY CONSIDERATIONS FOR REMOTE MONITORING MANAGEMENT

This review reinforces that an organized model for RM clinics is required to support the guidelines for RM follow-up of CIEDs. A primary nursing model may be ideal and most feasible in practice. When establishing an RM clinic as part of an EP practice, there are several considerations for setting up the organizational model, data management, and workflow. Additionally, there are important considerations for vendors supporting the management of CIED data and policymakers involved in establishing guidelines for CIED management and data standards (**Table 3**).

SUMMARY

The increase in number and complexity of CIEDs and standards for RM follow-up has led to a need for more guidance on organizational models for RM. This review provides an overview of the literature assessing RM clinic models, current recommendations, and considerations for RM management. Observations from current research suggests that the primary nursing model may be optimal, most importantly with a dedicated CIED team consisting of CIED certified nurse(s) and supervising EP(s) to manage CIED data, and to act as the first filter for transmission data. Challenges for the management of RM data include multiple manufacturers, lack of standardization and interoperability, abundance of data and alerts, and transmission failures. Additionally, patient engagement and assessing their needs are important parts of the workflow. A key barrier to the uptake of RM is lack of reimbursement models. When implementing an RM clinic, key considerations are structuring the CIED team with defined roles and responsibilities, use of middleware to organize the data and help with administrative tasks, and improved efforts to support and provide education to patients.

While a thorough search of the literature was performed for this review, it was not systematic and thus the articles cited do not necessarily represent an exhaustive review of the topic. The majority of articles discussed in this review are from Western European countries and the United States. Therefore a global perspective of RM clinics is not represented. More research may be warranted to understand the role of RM from a global perspective. The content in this article represents viewpoints of the authors and do not represent those of Parkview Health or any other organization.

CLINICS CARE POINTS

- The abundance of data from RM of CIEDs is growing as a result of increased number of implants
- The future of RM management involves leveraging advanced technologies to assist with integration and interoperability and optimizing reports for clinical decision making
- Management of RM data requires a robust organizational model that takes into consideration the workflows for managing data and for patient care

ACKNOWLEDGEMENTS

The authors would like to acknowledge Sarah Ellsworth-Hoffman, MLS for assisting in the literature search and Dr. Gerald Serwer, MD for review of the article.

DISCLOSURE

Dr M. Mirro reports grants from the Agency for Healthcare Research and Quality and Medtronic PLC, consulting fees/honoraria from McKesson and Zoll Medical Corporation; and nonpublic equity/stock interest in Murj, Inc/Viscardia. Dr M. Mirro's relationships with academia include serving as a trustee of Indiana University. Dr. Tammy Toscos reports grants from Biotronik, Inc, Medtronic PLC, Janssen Scientific Affairs, and iRhythm Technologies, Inc. Ms. Daley reports grants from Medtronic, PLC. All other authors have nothing to disclose.

REFERENCES

1. Piccini JP, Mittal S, Snell J, et al. Impact of remote monitoring on clinical events and associated health care utilization: a nationwide assessment. Heart Rhythm 2016;13(12):2279–86.

2. Wilkoff BL, Auricchio A, Brugada J, et al. HRS/EHRA expert consensus on the monitoring of cardiovascular implantable electronic devices (CIEDs): description of techniques, indications, personnel, frequency and ethical considerations: developed in partnership with the Heart Rhythm Society (HRS) and the European Heart Rhythm Association (EHRA); and in collaboration with the American College of Cardiology (ACC), the American Heart Association (AHA), the European Society of Cardiology (ESC), the Heart Failure Association of ESC (HFA), and the Heart Failure Society of America (HFSA). Endorsed by the Heart Rhythm Society, the European Heart Rhythm Association (a registered branch of the ESC), the American College of Cardiology, the American Heart Association. Europace 2008;10(6):707–25.

3. Marinskis G, van Erven L, Bongiorni MG, et al. Practices of cardiac implantable electronic device follow-up: results of the European Heart Rhythm Association survey. Europace 2012;14(3):423–5.

4. Palmisano P, Melissano D, Zanotto G, et al. Change in the use of remote monitoring of cardiac implantable electronic devices in Italian clinical practice over a 5-year period: results of two surveys promoted by the AIAC (Italian Association of Arrhythmology and Cardiac Pacing). J Cardiovasc Med 2020;21(4):305–14.

5. Kelly SE, Campbell D, Duhn LJ, et al. Remote monitoring of cardiovascular implantable electronic devices in Canada: survey of patients and device healthcare professionals. CJC Open 2021;1;3(4):391–9.

6. Ricci RP, Morichelli L. Patient satisfaction, clinic workflow, and efficiency. In: Steinberg JS, Varma N, editors. Remote monitoring: implantable devices and ambulatory ECG. Philadelphia: Wolters Kluwer; 2020. p. 76–82.

7. HRS COVID-19 task force update: April 15, 2020. Available at: https://www.hrsonline.org/COVID19-Challenges-Solutions/hrs-covid-19-task-force-update-april-15-2020. Accessed November 24, 2020.

8. Mittal S, Movsowitz C, Varma N. The modern EP practice: EHR and remote monitoring. Cardiol Clin 2014;32(2):239–52.

9. Slotwiner D, Varma N, Akar JG, et al. HRS Expert Consensus Statement on remote interrogation and monitoring for cardiovascular implantable electronic devices. Heart Rhythm 2015;12(7):e69–100.

10. Varma N. Remote monitoring of patients with CIEDs: what do the guidelines say. In: Steinberg JS, VN, editors. Remote monitoring: implantable devices and ambulatory ECG. Philadelphia: Wolters Kluwer; 2020. p. 99–103.

11. Husser D, Christoph Geller J, Taborsky M, et al. Remote monitoring and clinical outcomes: details on information flow and workflow in the IN-TIME

study. Eur Heart J Qual Care Clin Outcomes 2019; 5(2):136–44.

12. Hidefjäll P. Drivers and barriers for implementing remote monitoring of patients with cardiac implantable electronic devices in Sweden–a mixed methods study. Int J Healthc 2020;13(1):1–11.

13. Boriani G, Burri H, Mantovani LG, et al. Device therapy and hospital reimbursement practices across European countries: a heterogeneous scenario. Europace 2011;13(suppl_2):ii59–65.

14. Müller A, Goette A, Perings C, et al. Potential role of telemedical service centers in managing remote monitoring data transmitted daily by cardiac implantable electronic devices: results of the early detection of cardiovascular events in device patients with heart failure (detecT-Pilot) study. Telemed J E Health 2013;19(6):460–6.

15. Vogtmann T, Stiller S, Marek A, et al. Workload and usefulness of daily, centralized home monitoring for patients treated with CIEDs: results of the MoniC (Model Project Monitor Centre) prospective multicentre study. Europace 2013;15(2):219–26.

16. Ricci RP, Morichelli L, D'Onofrio A, et al. Manpower and outpatient clinic workload for remote monitoring of patients with cardiac implantable electronic devices: data from the HomeGuide Registry. J Cardiovasc Electrophysiol 2014;25(11):1216–23.

17. Guédon-Moreau L, Finat L, Boulé S, et al. Validation of an organizational management model of remote implantable cardioverter-defibrillator monitoring alerts. Circ Cardiovasc Qual Outcomes 2015;8(4):403–12.

18. Dario C, Delise P, Gubian L, et al. Large controlled observational study on remote monitoring of pacemakers and implantable cardiac defibrillators: a clinical, economic, and organizational evaluation. Interact J Med Res 2016;5(1):e4.

19. Giannola G, Torcivia R, Farulla RA, et al. Outsourcing the remote management of cardiac implantable electronic devices: medical care quality improvement project. JMIR Cardio 2019;3(2):e9815.

20. Zanotto G, D'Onofrio A, Della Bella P, et al. Organizational model and reactions to alerts in remote monitoring of cardiac implantable electronic devices: a survey from the Home Monitoring Expert Alliance project. Clin Cardiol 2019;42(1):76–83.

21. Zanotto G, Melissano D, Baccillieri S, et al. Intrahospital organizational model of remote monitoring data sharing, for a global management of patients with cardiac implantable electronic devices: a document of the Italian Association of Arrhythmology and Cardiac Pacing. J Cardiovasc Med 2020;21(3): 171–81.

22. Lucà F, Cipolletta L, Di Fusco SA, et al. Remote monitoring: doomed to let down or an attractive promise? Int J Cardiol Heart Vasc 2019;24:100380.

23. Slotwiner D. Electronic health records and implantable devices: new paradigms and efficiencies. In: Steinberg JS, Varma N, editors. Remote monitoring: implantable devices and ambulatory ECG. Philadelphia: Wolters Kluwer; 2020. p. 83–8.

24. Meyer A. Going paperless in the device clinic: automating via an Implantable Cardiac Device Observation workflow. EP Lab Dig 2020;20(11). Available at: https://www.eplabdigest.com/going-paperless-device-clinic-automating-implantable-device-cardiac-observation-workflow.

25. de Ruvo E, Sciarra L, Martino AM, et al. A prospective comparison of remote monitoring systems in implantable cardiac defibrillators: potential effects of frequency of transmissions. J Interv Card Electrophysiol 2016;45(1):81–90.

26. Afzal MR, Mease J, Koppert T, et al. Incidence of false-positive transmissions during remote rhythm monitoring with implantable loop recorders. Heart Rhythm 2020;17(1):75–80.

27. O'Shea CJ, Middeldorp ME, Hendriks JM, et al. Remote monitoring alert burden: an analysis of transmission in> 26,000 patients. JACC Clin Electrophysiol 2021;7(2):226–34.

28. Ploux S, Varma N, Strik M, et al. Optimizing implantable cardioverter-defibrillator remote monitoring: a practical guide. JACC Clin Electrophysiol 2017; 3(4):315–28.

29. Cronin EM, Ching EA, Varma N, et al. Remote monitoring of cardiovascular devices: a time and activity analysis. Heart Rhythm 2012;9(12):1947–51.

30. Burri H, Heidbüchel H, Jung W, et al. Remote monitoring: a cost or an investment? Europace 2011; 13(suppl_2):ii44–8.

31. Srivatsa UN, Joy KC, Zhang XJ, et al. Patient perception of the remote versus clinic visits for interrogation of implantable cardioverter defibrillators. Crit Pathw Cardiol 2020;19(1):22–5.

32. Timmermans I, Meine M, Szendey I, et al. Remote monitoring of implantable cardioverter defibrillators: patient experiences and preferences for follow-up. Pacing Clin Electrophysiol 2019;42(2):120–9.

33. Skov MB, Johansen PG, Skov CS, et al. No news is good news: remote monitoring of implantable cardioverter-defibrillator patients. Paper presented at: Proceedings of the 33rd annual ACM conference on human factors in computing systems 2015 Apr 18 (pp. 827–836).

34. Petersen HH, Larsen MCJ, Nielsen OW, et al. Patient satisfaction and suggestions for improvement of remote ICD monitoring. J Interv Card Electrophysiol 2012;34(3):317–24.

35. Safarikova I, Bulava A, Hajek P. Remote monitoring of implantable cardioverters defibrillators: a comparison of acceptance between octogenarians and younger patients. J Geriatr Cardiol 2020;17(7):417.

36. Freedman A, Nicolle J. Social isolation and loneliness: the new geriatric giants: approach for primary care. Can Fam Physician 2020;66(3):176–82.

37. Laurent G, Amara W, Mansourati J, et al. Role of patient education in the perception and acceptance of home monitoring after recent implantation of cardioverter defibrillators: the EDUCAT study. Arch Cardiovasc Dis 2014;107(10):508–18.

38. Andersen TO, Nielsen KD, Moll J, et al. Unpacking telemonitoring work: workload and telephone calls to patients in implanted cardiac device care. Int J Med Inform 2019;129:381–7.

39. Al-Khatib SM, Mi X, Wilkoff BL, et al. Follow-up of patients with new cardiovascular implantable electronic devices: are experts' recommendations implemented in routine clinical practice? Circ Arrhythm Electrophysiol 2013;6(1):108–16.

40. Varma N, Piccini JP, Snell J, et al. The relationship between level of adherence to automatic wireless remote monitoring and survival in pacemaker and defibrillator patients. J Am Coll Cardiol 2015; 65(24):2601–10.

41. Mantini N, Borne RT, Varosy PD, et al. Use of cell phone adapters is associated with reduction in disparities in remote monitoring of cardiac implantable electronic devices. J Interv Card Electrophysiol 2021;60:469–75.

42. Rosenfeld LE, Patel AS, Ajmani VB, et al. Compliance with remote monitoring of ICDS/CRTDS in a real-world population. Pacing Clin Electrophysiol 2014;37(7):820–7.

43. Liljeroos M, Thylén I, Strömberg A. Patients' and nurses' experiences and perceptions of remote monitoring of implantable cardiac defibrillators in heart failure: cross-sectional, descriptive, mixed methods study. J Med Internet Res 2020;22(9): e19550.

44. Crossley GH, Boyle A, Vitense H, et al. The CONNECT (Clinical Evaluation of Remote Notification to Reduce Time to Clinical Decision) trial: the value of wireless remote monitoring with automatic clinician alerts. J Am Coll Cardiol 2011;57(10):1181–9.

45. Halimi F, Cantù F. Remote monitoring for active cardiovascular implantable electronic devices: a European survey. Europace 2010;12(12):1778–80.

46. Schoenfeld MH, Reynolds DW, et al. Sophisticated remote implantable cardioverter-defibrillator follow-up: A status report. Pacing Clin Electrophysiol 2005;28(3):235–40.

47. Medtronic expands technology solutions to help physicians manage cardiac device data; improved access to data reinforces medtronic leadership in patient management. Available at: https://www.businesswire.com/news/home/20050504005752/en/Medtronic-Expands-Technology-Solutions-Physicians-Manage-Cardiac#:%7E:text=Medtronic%20also%20announced%20the%20release,System%2C%20its%202005%20First%20Edition. Accessed December 21, 2020.

48. Biundo E, Lanctin D, Rosemas SC, et al. Vendor-neutral clinic management software use is associated with time savings for remote monitoring. Circ Cardiovasc Qual Outcomes 2020;13(Suppl_1): A287.

49. Daley CN, Chen EM, Roebuck AE, et al. Providing patients with implantable cardiac device data through a personal health record: a qualitative study. Appl Clin Inform 2017;8(4):1106.

50. Mirro M, Daley C, Wagner S, et al. Delivering remote monitoring data to patients with implantable cardioverter-defibrillators: does medium matter? Pacing Clin Electrophysiol 2018;41(11):1526–35.

51. Ahmed R, Toscos T, Ghahari RR, et al. Visualization of cardiac implantable electronic device data for older adults using participatory design. Appl Clin Inform 2019;10(4):707.

52. Daley C, Ghahari RR, Drouin M, et al. Involving patients as key stakeholders in the design of cardiovascular implantable electronic device data dashboards: implications for patient care. Heart Rhythm O2 2020;1(2):136–46.

53. Toscos T, Daley C, Wagner S, et al. Patient responses to daily cardiac resynchronization therapy device data: a pilot trial assessing a novel patient-centered digital dashboard in everyday life. Cardiovascular Digital Health Journal 2020;1(2):97–106.

54. Daley C, Cornet V, Patekar G, et al. Uncertainty Management Among Older Adults with Heart Failure: Responses to Receiving Implanted Device Data using a Fictitious Scenario Interview Method. Paper presented at: Proceedings of the International Symposium on Human Factors and Ergonomics in Health Care2019 Sep (Vol. 8, No. 1, pp. 127–100).

55. Cohen IG, Gerke S, Kramer DB. Ethical and legal implications of remote monitoring of medical devices. Milbank Q 2020;98(4):1257–89.

56. Daley C, Toscos T, Mirro M. Data integration and interoperability for patient-centered remote monitoring of cardiovascular implantable electronic devices. Bioengineering 2019;6(1):25.

Cybersecurity of Cardiovascular Implantable Electronic Devices and Remote Programming

David J. Slotwiner, MD, FHRS[a],*, Kenneth P. Hoyme, MSEE[b], Sudar Shields, MSEE[c]

KEYWORDS

- Cardiac implantable electronic devices • Remote reprogramming • Cybersecurity
- Asymmetric encryption • Chain of trust • End-to-end secure messaging • Coordinated disclosure

KEY POINTS

- Given enough time and resources, a skilled cybersecurity intruder is likely to find a vulnerability in any system, providing an entry point and enabling the intruder to hack the system. One goal of cybersecurity is to make it sufficiently difficult to hack a system that an adversary would find the target a poor return on their resource and effort investment, and move on to a more vulnerable target.
- The ability to remotely reprogram a cardiac implantable electronic device (CIED) and the ability to remotely install software or firmware updates would reduce the need for in-office visits and could provide a mechanism to rapidly deploy important software or firmware updates.
- Consideration will be needed to determine which parameters should be remotely programmable, and whether boundaries should be placed on these parameters for patient safety. The setting (home or medical office) in which remote reprogramming occurs may influence which parameters should be reprogrammable.
- The challenges of implementing remote reprogramming of cardiac implantable electronic devices are no longer technical. Using asymmetric cryptography, sophisticated end-to-end secure communication protocols and hardware accelerators, the resources required to identify and take advantage of a cybersecurity vulnerability of a single CIED would be very significant and likely well beyond the gain that an intruder would deem worthwhile.

INTRODUCTION

Remote monitoring of implantable pacemakers, defibrillators and subcutaneous cardiac rhythm monitors has become the standard of care, providing early notification of clinically actionable events including arrhythmias, lead or device malfunction, reducing shocks, and avoiding hospitalizations.[1] The Heart Rhythm Society's 2015 Expert Consensus Statement on Remote Interrogation and Monitoring of Cardiovascular Implantable Electronic Devices (CIEDs) recommends at least 1 in-person office evaluation per year. The purpose of this evaluation is to provide an opportunity to make routine programming adjustments, install any nonurgent software or firmware updates, and give the patient and provider an opportunity to address any changes in health conditions and any questions that may have arisen. As telehealth has now become widely accepted by patients and

a Division of Cardiology, New York Presbyterian Queens, School of Population Health Sciences, Weill Cornell Medicine, 56-45 Main Street, Flushing, NY 11355, USA; b Global Product Cybersecurity, Boston Scientific, 4100 Hamline Avenue North, St Paul, MN 55112, USA; c Product Security Systems Architect, Global Product Cybersecurity, Boston Scientific, 4100 Hamline Avenue North, St Paul, MN 55112, USA
* Corresponding author. New York Presbyterian Queens, 56-45 Main Street, Flushing, NY 11355, USA
E-mail address: djs2001@med.cornell.edu

Card Electrophysiol Clin 13 (2021) 499–508
https://doi.org/10.1016/j.ccep.2021.04.007

providers, largely due to the COVID-19 pandemic, the advantages of delivering care remotely are becoming increasingly appreciated by patients and providers. Remote reprograming of CIEDs, including the ability to provide software and firmware updates, could significantly increase the ability of clinicians to manage patients with CIEDs without requiring in-office visits. The annual in-office visit could be replaced with a telehealth visit, and any reprogramming changes or software and firmware updates could be pushed to the devices without waiting for the patient's annual visit. The concerns surrounding remote reprogramming have never been about technical capability. Rather, they have focused on practical considerations regarding patient safety and concerns that remote reprogramming could introduce opportunities that might attract cybersecurity hackers. As more care is delivered remotely, and with advancements in microchip that now permit asymmetric cryptography and sophisticated end-to-end secure communication protocols without significant power consumption, the addition of remote reprogramming capabilities to CIEDs is likely to proceed.

CYBERSECURITY VULNERABILITIES OF MEDICAL DEVICES

Given enough time and resources, a skilled cyber-security intruder is likely to find a vulnerability in any system, providing an entry point and enabling the intruder to hack the system. Most recently, this has been demonstrated by the hack of SolarWinds software, which allowed what appears to be the Russian government to pierce the cybersecurity defenses of the US government as well as thousands of companies across the United States, including FireEye, the widely recognized premier company focused on cybersecurity.[2]

Given the interconnected nature of our modern world, with the Internet of things touching virtually every aspect of daily life, one goal of cybersecurity is to make it sufficiently difficult to hack a system that an adversary would find the target a poor return on their resource and effort investment, and move on to a more vulnerable target. On August 25, 2016, Muddy Waters LLC released to the public a report from the cybersecurity research firm MedSec that claimed to show that St. Jude Medical CIEDs were vulnerable to cybersecurity hacking via the Merlin@Home transmitter, and that a skilled intruder could cause a defibrillator to deliver an unnecessary shock, and/or result in premature battery depletion. MedSec publicly noted that they focused on St. Jude's devices, as they were easier to exploit.

This claim was greeted with a mixed response: fear from the public; confusion from the medical

community; and panic and opportunity from the investment world. To date, the public's concern about medical devices and cybersecurity were primarily guided by a 2012 episode of the popular TV series Homeland during which a US Vice President candidate is assassinated by a hacker who reprograms his pacemaker. It should be noted that this fictional episode assumed that activation of the high rates used for inducing arrhythmia are possible from modern pacemakers: most have safety features that would prevent this. In 2001, former Vice President Dick Cheney also requested that wireless functionality of his Medtronic implantable cardioverter defibrillator (ICD) be disabled for security purposes. The medical community, including manufacturers and the US Food and Drug Administration had been focused on the security risks of medical devices directly connected to a network, as the highest risk devices. CIEDS, which were only connected to approved accessories were thought to have managed safety and security risk to an acceptable level. The investment community was focused on the sale of St. Jude Medical to Abbott, with short-selling investment firms such as Muddy Waters LLC poised to reap significant profits if the value of St. Jude Medical plummeted. Beyond an interesting story, this event brought to light how unprepared the medical community was to evaluate and manage a potential cybersecurity vulnerability, and the fundamental differences between cybersecurity threats in comparison to device or lead malfunctions and recalls with which the clinical community was quite familiar. It also highlights a key cybersecurity issue for remote reprogramming to ensure that only instructions/commands received by a CIED from an authenticated, trustworthy source are executed.

The St. Jude Medical Story

Details explaining MedSec's claim that St. Jude Medical CIEDs were vulnerable to hacking have been summarized for a lay audience by cybersecurity researcher Matthew Green, a cryptographer and professor at Johns Hopkins University.[3] Professor Green was part of a team of independent cybersecurity researchers hired by the law firm defending MedSec against St. Jude Medical's (now owned by Abbott) defamation law suit. His team confirmed that it was possible to reprogram a St. Jude Medical ICD using only the hardware contained within a Merlin@Home communicator and to disable therapy and/or issue commands to deliver a high-power shock. The researchers first examined the programming code on a St. Jude Medical programmer and were able to identify the portion of the code responsible for authenticating the programmer to the implanted device, and for encrypting and issuing programming commands to the implantable device. Next, they installed a new package of software containing these instructions onto a Merlin@Home device. Then they were able to issue reprogramming commands from the Merlin @Home device which were verified by interrogating the ICD with a St. Jude Medical programmer. The fact that these steps were easily exploitable indicated significant security concerns at 3 levels.

As Matthew Green explains, the fact that it was easy to identify the portion of the computer code on the St. Jude programmer responsible for issuing commands is unusual. Typically, steps are taken to obfuscate sensitive portions of computer code for just this reason. Furthermore, they were able to determine that commands issued by the programmer were authenticated by the implanted device using only a universal 3-byte (24-bit) authentication tag that had to be present and correct with each command issued to the device. This relatively short tag might have made it difficult enough to deter potential hackers if the tag were created using a secure cryptographic function and a fresh secret key that cannot be predicted. But instead, St. Jude Medical used a "key table" hard coded in the software of the programmer. Therefore, anyone who had access to a St. Jude programmer and the technical skills could download the table and gain the ability to calculate the correct authentication tags needed to produce commands that the implanted device would then execute. In addition, a nonstandard application of the Rivest-Shamir-Adelman (RSA) algorithm that also involved the use of weak, hardcoded, nonstandard keys in the protocol (see asymmetric encryption). The final vulnerability MedSec illuminated was the fact that St. Jude Medical CIEDs would accept reprogramming codes sent via radiofrequency communication (distance of several feet) without first requiring communication via inductive telemetry (requiring the programming wand to be placed over the device). Requiring a reprogramming session to be initiated by inductive telemetry necessitates the individual interrogating/reprogramming the CIED to be in very close physical contact with the patient, providing an important measure of security.

REMOTE PROGRAMMING: SPECIAL CONSIDERATIONS
Patient Safety and Practical Considerations

When considering remote reprogramming of CIEDs, many topics that we take for granted when reprogramming is performed in the office become much more complex. These include considering whether all programmable parameters should be remotely reprogrammable, should there be safety boundaries on ranges of settings (eg, minimum heart rates), how and when patients should be informed, how and when patient or caregiver consent should be obtained, should there be different categories of remote reprogramming for patients who are at home versus those who in a medical setting with remote reprogramming from an electrophysiologist, and should there be a "time-out" period during which a patient can reverse the reprogramming if they feel unwell?

Present implantable cardiac rhythm monitors manufactured by Boston Scientific have no restrictions on which parameters can be remotely reprogrammed, and the changes can occur without the patient being informed. But these devices serve non–life-sustaining diagnostic roles and have no therapeutic capabilities. Pacemakers and ICDs that serve life-sustaining functions raise much more complicated considerations.

Which parameters should be reprogrammable?
Most CIED parameters never require reprogramming following the initial device implant, and current generation CIEDs uniformly have the ability to monitor and auto-adjust pacing output. It would be useful to be able to temporarily suspend tachytherapies for ICD patients presenting for surgical procedures, MRIs, or other medical interventions that might interfere with the device's function. This would also be helpful for the rare ICD patient whose device's tachytherapies were inadvertently left inactive following a procedure. Reprogramming the upper and/or lower pacing rates, or rate-adaptive parameters could be helpful for patients with symptomatic bradycardia or chronotropic incompetence. Many physiologic alerts provided by present generation CIEDs are programmed in the device and being able to optimize these remotely according to the individual patient's indications could greatly alleviate the burden of alerts received by the remote monitoring facility.

Placing safety boundaries to limit the reprogramming could mitigate the risk of causing harm. For example, limiting the ability to inhibit pacing completely, or check atrial pacing thresholds in atrial only pacing mode could prevent a pacemaker-dependent patient from being inadvertently placed in a dangerous situation. Similarly, patient harm could be mitigated by restricting the remote programming of parameters whose configurations are shown by research to be proarrhythmic or a drain on the implantable device's battery.

Another safety measure that could be used would be to require a patient to confirm or validate a reprogrammed parameter within a short time, or the parameter would revert back to its original value. For example, a pacemaker's lower rate could be reprogrammed from 60 to 50 beats per minute and the patient would need to acknowledge this by pressing an authenticated button on their remote monitoring application within a specified time interval or the parameter would revert back to 60 beats per minute.

Should patients be informed?

In a medical setting, patients know when their pacemaker or defibrillator is being interrogated because, by safety design, an inductive telemetry wand must first be placed within inches of the device to establish communication. Radiofrequency communication then takes over, allowing the wand to be removed and the interrogation and reprogramming can be performed from a distance of several feet. During this session the patients know and implicitly consent to the interaction. Occasionally, in addition to the interrogation and reprogramming, software or firmware updates are installed to patch cybersecurity vulnerabilities or other functional updates.

Remote reprogramming could be used to adjust pacing or rate-response therapies to alleviate patients' symptoms, but most likely the real benefit would be for reprogramming parameters of which the patient is unaware. Cybersecurity and other software updates, such as those received periodically by our smartphones and computers, would be a potentially powerful way to quickly and securely address an implantable vulnerability, or to roll out security and safety enhancements. Yet there is always a small risk that a software or firmware update will have an unanticipated deleterious effect, shortening battery life, interfering with routine device function, or permanently disabling an implantable device in the worst-case. An unexpected failure for a smartphone is quite different from an unexpected failure of a CIED.

Informing patients before CIED reprogramming would delay and complicate the process of reprogramming, and some may elect not to receive what could be important safety updates. Nevertheless, given the high stakes of CIED function, it is difficult to conceive of denying patients this basic right.

Environment

Considerations for remote reprogramming are different if a patient is located at home versus in an observed medical environment, and this might factor into which parameters should be reprogrammable based on patient location. In rural areas, patients could travel to their local primary care physician and then establish a remote programming session with their electrophysiologist hundreds of miles away. A nurse or technician could provide assistance and observe the patient and communicate with the remote electrophysiologist to relay symptoms or untoward effects. Under these circumstances, there might not be a need to place limits on which parameters could be reprogrammed.

Requiring inductive telemetry in order to initiate "safe environment" or "break glass" remote reprogramming use cases would allow remote programming to inherit a similar proximity-based implicit trust model as that implemented in the programming use cases in prior generation CIEDs. However, new generation Bluetooth-enabled CIEDs that are programmed using mobile-based clinician apps could potentially run into usability or increased footprint (can-size) issues if inductive telemetry circuitry is required for remote programming. A zero-trust architecture with a well-designed and well-implemented public key infrastructure (PKI) (**Table 1**) that uses end-to-end encryption cryptographic message authentication, and code signing can be an effective alternative to inductive telemetry. There is also increasing awareness of the limitations suffered by proximity-based implicit trust models when subjected to social engineering or physical attacks similar to those observed against early contactless payment cards when there was news coverage about criminals physically tapping card skimmers over victims' pockets in crowded public spaces such as concerts and trains.

Finally, because reliable auto-detection of the patient's current environment (home vs clinical setting) is not trivial, the scenario described here may necessitate an extra authorization step from the attending local clinician (present at the patient's location) before the activation of remote programming features that are only available in a clinical setting.[4]

Technical Considerations

The security vulnerability exposed by Muddy Waters Research LLC and MedSec illustrates the fundamental challenge that needs to be overcome by safe and secure remote reprogramming solutions. It is essential that the implanted CIED be able to verify that any command it executes originates from a trusted source. This source could be the patient's health care team, the CIED manufacturer, or (in limited scenarios) the patient's authorized caregiver or the patient themselves. The

Table 1
Key terms of computer cryptography

Terminology	Definition
Encryption	The process of converting information or data into unintelligible text or data to prevent unauthorized access.
Key	A string of random bits that encrypts or decrypts data.
Symmetric encryption	A type of encryption in which only one key is used to both encrypt and decrypt electronic information.
Asymmetric encryption	A type of encryption in which the encryption key and the corresponding decryption key are different. The private and public keys are mathematically related, but there is no way to practically derive one from the other.
Private key	The key used in asymmetric encryption protocols to encrypt and sign data.
Public key	The key used in asymmetric encryption protocols to decrypt data and confirm authenticity of the source.
Chain of trust	A concept in computer security. A chain of trust is established by validating each component of hardware and software from the end entity up to the root certificate. It is intended to ensure that only trusted software and hardware can be used while still retaining flexibility.
End-to-end encryption	A system of communication in which only the sender and intended final recipient can decrypt the data. Any intermediary systems in the communication serve as simply pass-through devices with no ability to decipher the data.
PKI	Public Key Infrastructure. The framework and services that provide for the generation, production, distribution, control, accounting, and destruction of public key certificates (or public-private key pairs). Components include the personnel, policies, processes, server platforms, software, and workstations used for the purpose of administering certificates and public-private key pairs, including the ability to issue, maintain, recover, and revoke public key certificates.
Authenticity	The property that data originated from its purported source.
Integrity	A property whereby data has not been altered in an unauthorized manner since it was created, transmitted, or stored.
Hardware accelerator	Micro processing chip (hardware) dedicated to quickly execute a specific computer command with very little power consumption.

importance of verifying that data are coming from a trusted and authorized source is not unique to CIEDs, and in fact has become ubiquitous as we have become dependent on the Internet. Banking, shopping, email, and countless other activities performed across the Internet all require us to be able to send data securely and to have systems in place that make it possible for the receiving system to verify the authenticity of the incoming data. PKI and code signing enabled by asymmetric cryptography, and end-to-end secure messaging have become the tools of choice to address this challenge. These are enabled by hardware-based root-of-trust (eg, secure crypto-processors in Hardware Security Modules, Trust Platform Modules, and smartcards) implemented in the backend infrastructure and in non-implantable elements in the CIED system. The CIEDs themselves are resistant to hardware attacks in their operational state by dint of the CIEDs' location inside the patient. Until recently, the power requirements of microchips prohibited consideration of use of asymmetric cryptography in CIEDs. Fortunately, this is no longer a limiting factor.

Trust

An essential requirement for the safe and secure programming of a CIED is the concept of trust. In the clinic, this trust is established by the presence of trained nurses and physicians with access to the specialized equipment used for programming. However, when the programming is done remotely, trust must be managed by cryptographic means.

Two key elements of trust are authenticity and integrity (see **Table 1**). Authenticity is the assurance that the programming commands came from an authorized source. Integrity is the assurance that the commands have not been modified in an unauthorized manner.

Cryptographic authenticity is usually implemented using public keys or digital certificates that can be used by the recipient to confirm the source's identity. Cryptographic authenticity is also used to validate the trustworthiness of code in secure boot implementations. Cryptographic integrity can be implemented using digital signatures, message authentication codes, or authenticated encryption that ensures that an attacker who modifies or falsifies programming commands without having the credentials used to sign authentic commands cannot produce a correct signature that will be accepted by the CIED.

On the Internet, trust can be managed through an approach referred to as "chain of trust." Chain of trust is about authenticating each element in the chain through the previously authenticated element in the same chain using certificates signed by previous elements (called intermediary authorities) in the chain all the way up to the root-of-trust (called the certificate authority). Verifying the chain of trust is possible in the offline mode, when access to the Internet connection is not available. So, this concept is also conducive to CIED use cases. Chain of trust requires asymmetric cryptography, so it requires the CIED to perform complex operations that have the potential to affect power consumption and essential performance. However, dedicated cryptographic processors are now possible in CIED hardware architectures. In addition, optimizations on the chain-of-trust concept can prevent adverse impacts to the CIED's battery life. For example, the intermediary certificates can be eliminated in CIED PKI implementations if the manufacturer provisions their own root key pairs. This introduces additional onus on the manufacturer to manage and secure their own PKI infrastructure, but allows for less complexity on the CIED. This elimination also allows root public keys to be installed in the CIEDs in place of digital certificates, because there are not any intermediary entities to validate.

End-to-end secure messaging, also known as encryption (E2EE), is a proven zero-trust concept that allows 2 entities to securely communicate over hostile communication channels. The keys used to encrypt and authenticate messages are only known to the 2 entities. The messages are encrypted and integrity-protected by the source entity, and any intermediate devices through which the messages travel are mere pass-through with no knowledge of the message contents. The receiving entity is able to authenticate and decrypt the messages, and thus able to detect any attempts by intermediate devices or the communication channel to tamper with the end-to-end secured messages. End-to-end secure messaging, thus enables a manufacturer's back-end services to securely communicate with the manufacturer's CIEDs with all the other devices (eg, mobile apps and embedded devices like bedside patient monitors) and communication channels (eg, Bluetooth, WiFi, Ethernet data links) in the communication pathway serving as mere pass-through data bridges. The manufacturer's server uses a private key (described as follows) to sign CIED firmware updates, and the CIED is installed with the server's public key. In this system, an intermediary is not able to undetectably modify the firmware image. Similarly, the manufacturer's sever uses end-to-end private keys provisioned to a specific CIED to encrypt and integrity-protect the CIED's remote programming commands. The CIED is the only other entity that has knowledge of these end-to-end private keys, so there is no risk of tampered commands being executed. This is particularly important if personal mobile phones are to be used as pass-through devices to allow remote communication with the CIED.

Note that in all of these cases, the CIED must be the enforcer of trust. Before longer-range radiofrequency (RF) protocols were added, only extremely near-field inductive links were used in CIED communications, and that physical proximity led to implicit trust from the CIED to the programmer. To save power, complex computations were done in the programmer and the results trusted by the CIED, because the programmer software and the CIED were tested together to the highest regulatory classification. Because longer-range RF protocols (including Bluetooth) can be manipulated more easily from a distance, it is no longer appropriate to implicitly trust an external device. The CIED must have the capability to execute the cryptographic protocols to establish trust. Proximity-based activation may be used in such a cryptography-based trust model as an additional trust factor, but it is no longer sufficient as the sole trust factor or authentication factor.

Encryption

Encryption refers to a process of converting information (called "plaintext") into a form ("ciphertext") that prevents unauthorized access. Converting the ciphertext back into plaintext requires that the receiver have a "key" that instructs the receiving system how to decrypt it. The challenge is managing the key so that it remains secure and known only to authorized receivers.

Symmetric-Key Encryption

Symmetric-key encryption algorithms use identical keys for the source and the destination. This requires that the sending and receiving systems share identical keys. A common example is the Advanced Encryption Standard. Symmetric algorithms tend to be efficient to execute in software.

The challenge with symmetric encryption is the secure management of the key(s). In the absence of other secure means such as asymmetric cryptography, there needs to be a shared secret or an independent (out-of-band) channel to ensure that both communicating endpoints derive the same key. Shared secrets can be built in at manufacturing time and stored securely, so they never have to be exchanged over the network. Or an out-of-band communications channel such as an inductive telemetry session could be used. Plans need to be made in the initial design, as in the absence of asymmetric crypto capabilities and out-of-band communication channels, it is difficult to securely distribute symmetric keys after a large fleet of devices are already in use in the field.

Although more complex, having a separate symmetric key for each CIED is more secure than using a common key for every device. Common keys are the machine-to-machine equivalent to a universal password, and if that single key is exposed, the trust mechanisms are at risk for all devices. For the same reason, symmetric keys used to secure a communication session should be resettable and preferably ephemeral, wherein a fresh session key is generated for each session through the active participation of both communicating entities.

A method needs to also be considered for how these keys are stored when in the devices that use them. Hardware encryption modules/chips (eg, Trusted Platform Module) can be used to shield the keys from being readable external to the module. If the key is stored in the CIED's nonvolatile storage, it does not provide any protection from an attacker who gets the CIED postexplant; but if that key is limited to that single device, it is less impactful to overall systems security. CIED cans have antitampering controls already implemented for safety reasons, so there are protections against unauthorized physical attacks on the CIED's nonvolatile storage. The CIED's location inside the patient during the device's operational phase also thwarts physical attacks on the CIED to acquire its keys.

Multiple symmetric keys may be stored in the CIED, including keys for remote programming, remote data collection, and even for firmware updating (code signing). Each key type embodies a level of privilege for accessing the CIED's information assets.

Using end-to-end trust mechanisms and using the intermediate device (eg, the smartphone) as a pass-through eliminates the need for the symmetric key to be installed in the intermediate device, limiting the threat surface for key discovery.

Asymmetric-Key Encryption

Asymmetric-key encryption are algorithms that use a key pair: a public key and a private or secret key. These keys are mathematically related, but there is no practical means to derive one from the other. The public key is exactly that: it can be provided to anyone, and on constantly connected Internet-based devices, there are means to discover public keys and even manage keys that have been "revoked" due to compromise of the private key. In addition, public keys can be signed by a higher certificate authority to generate digital certificates, thereby providing a means for 2 entities to authenticate each other, even if they do not know anything about each other and may have never had a prior encounter with each other. In other words, certificates eliminate the need to store in the authenticating device the identity information and authentication secrets such as passwords associated with the supplicant that is being authenticated. Authentication is possible as long as the authenticating device has the root certificate and the supplicant presents an unexpired certificate that was signed by the same certificate authority that corresponds to the root certificate.

Typical asymmetric-key algorithms include RSA (the typical standard for Internet TLS/SSL traffic), Diffie Hellman (used to securely exchange cryptographic keys over an open network), and Elliptical Curve Cryptography (ECC), which is more computationally efficient. However, asymmetric algorithms are computationally more complex to execute in software than symmetric algorithms.

Typical implementations of asymmetric cryptography and PKI in CIEDs use key pairs, instead of digital certificates and instead of a classic chain of trust that comprises intermediary entities. It is also possible to provision multiple key pairs in the CIED, including dedicated public-private key pairs for remote programming, remote data collection and firmware updating (code signing) respectively.

Similar to the discussion on symmetric-key encryption, the decision whether to use a common client authentication key pair for all CIEDs versus separate is relevant. However, if an attacker hacks a single CIED, they will only get the public keys for the server functions and the private keys used to authenticate the hacked CIED, which does not allow them to spoof commands that would become accepted by another CIED.

Energy considerations for implantable devices

CIEDs are designed to operate for up to 10 years or more on a single, nonrechargeable battery. Many techniques are implemented by manufacturers to meet this challenging requirement. This includes relatively slow clock speeds to save power. As a result, cryptographic algorithms written in software may not execute at an acceptable speed. Although symmetric algorithms are feasible, asymmetric algorithms may take several minutes to execute, making them impractical to use without hardware acceleration. CIED manufacturers, when designing the microchip architecture of a device, can purchase circuitry (hardware accelerator) developed specifically for executing a specific asymmetric encryption algorithm. This alleviates the primary circuitry of the device from the burden of performing the calculation using software, which would be both prohibitively slow and consume too much energy. ECC algorithms are more amenable to hardware implementation and are finding favor in battery-powered applications.

Energy optimization is also achievable in CIEDs by adopting existing best practices in cryptography wherein asymmetric cryptography is reserved for entity authentication, session authentication, symmetric key exchange, and firmware update digital signature validation, whereas symmetric keys are used for protecting the confidentiality, integrity, and message authenticity of control signals, such as programming commands.

Other energy considerations include protections against battery attacks, such as by enabling the CIEDs to monitor connection requests and active telemetry sessions for patterns that are known to be risky or anomalous (deviate from normal patterns) in other ways. The CIEDs would also need to enforce connection limits and session terminations, and may need to throttle or ignore connection requests (either temporarily or until inductive telemetry is activated) when established thresholds are met in these observed patterns.

IDENTIFYING AND DISCLOSING CYBERSECURITY VULNERABILITIES

Most cybersecurity vulnerabilities are not identified by individuals or groups with malicious intent. Most are brought to light by security researchers.

Once a potentially significant vulnerability is identified, it requires assessment by both the manufacturer and the Department of Homeland Security's Cybersecurity & Infrastructure Security Agency. The US Federal Bureau of Investigation becomes involved if potential criminal activity is suspected. If the suspected vulnerability is validated by the manufacturer and there is potential for patient harm, the US Food and Drug Administration must be notified. Involving the appropriate regulatory agencies along with the cybersecurity researcher(s) and manufacturer allows all parties to thoroughly evaluate and understand the vulnerability and develop a mitigation strategy. Once this is complete, a coordinated disclosure to public can take place: the manufacturer, regulatory agencies, and other stakeholders can inform the public of the vulnerability and at the same time provide guidance on the severity, likelihood of the vulnerability being exploited, consequences if it is exploited and mitigating strategies the public can use to minimize the risk.

The Muddy Waters LLC and MedSec announcement directly to the public illustrates an alternative pathway: a researcher or individual/group possibly with malicious intent may choose to go directly to the public to release the claim. Reasons for this may be based in a desire or financial interest in causing fear, chaos, or to affect the value of a company. Regardless of the motivation, it leaves the manufacturer, regulatory agencies and public scrambling to assess the validity of the claim, determine if mitigating steps should be taken immediately, and identifying a long-term strategy to eliminate the vulnerability. Although the FDA is reducing the barriers to fast response to cybersecurity corrections, they still expect the manufacturers to thoroughly test those corrections.

Research shows that only a small fraction of discovered vulnerabilities are observed to be exploited in the wild.[5,6] However, the number of vulnerabilities discovered annually are high and vulnerability scores like CVSS are not well-correlated with the likelihood of exploitation. Apart from limitations suffered by scoring metrics, there is also an element of subjectivity in which exploits get selected for use by cybercriminals and other adversaries. These factors render it hard to reliably and proactively identify whether a disclosed vulnerability will be exploited and the sheer volume of off-the-shelf software vulnerabilities disclosed every year introduce the potential for patients and their health care providers from becoming overwhelmed by individual vulnerability disclosures. Thus, an essential element of remote programming is a secure patching infrastructure that enables reliability, speed and periodicity in the testing and deployment of vulnerability fixes. This would allow conversations with patients to shift toward actionable solutions that periodically eliminate known risks in the form of readily available secure patches that can be opted-in by their health care providers or by the patients themselves.

THE ROLES OF ELECTROPHYSIOLOGIST AND ALLIED CARE PROFESSIONALS

Patients recognize that cybersecurity is beyond the expertise of their health care providers, yet they view their care providers as the best resource to guide them in managing cybersecurity vulnerabilities once identified. This was the unanimous consensus of patients who participated in the Heart Rhythm Society's Cybersecurity Leadership Summit.[7]

It is best practice to discuss cybersecurity with patients in advance of any specific vulnerability and to explain that a CIED, just like their smartphone, will likely require software or firmware updates that may include cybersecurity updates. If a specific vulnerability is identified, specific topics should be addressed:

- What might occur if the vulnerability is exploited?
- How technically difficult (likely) is it that an attacker could exploit the vulnerability?
- What can be done to mitigate the risk of the vulnerability being exploited?
- What is the benefit of the device versus the risk from the cybersecurity vulnerability?
- What is the long-term solution?

SUMMARY

The COVID-19 global pandemic has forced the public and health care providers to rapidly implement telehealth and other tools to assist in the management of health care delivered outside of the traditional medical establishment. This has helped identify both the advantages as well as the limitations of remote management with the present tools we have. The ability to remotely reprogram CIEDs is one example of a technology that could greatly extend the capabilities we have, potentially (in combination with telehealth) further reducing the need for in-office visits.

The challenges of implementing CIED remote reprogramming are no longer technical. Using asymmetric cryptography, sophisticated end-to-end secure communication protocols and hardware accelerators, the resources required to identify and take advantage of a cybersecurity vulnerability of a single CIED would be very significant and likely well beyond the gain that an intruder would deem worthwhile. Similarly, with hardware encryption modules, the ability of an intruder to spoof a CIED vendor's remote monitoring server is extremely remote.

Now the burden lies in considering how to implement remote reprogramming safely and effectively. This will require consideration of several factors including which parameters should be reprogrammable, whether there should be safety boundaries, whether patient location (home vs supervised medical environment) should be taken into consideration and most importantly what the role of the patient will be. The active role of reprogramming raises the stakes over simply remote monitoring. Developing clear and reliable patient communication strategies will be fundamental to its success.

CLINICS CARE POINTS

- Avoiding cybersecurity breaches requires vigilance from all members of the health care team.
- If a cybersecurity vulnerability of a cardiac implantable electronic device (CIEDs) becomes known, patients expect their health care provider to give them guidance on how to minimize their risk of harm. It is therefore important that health care providers familiarize themselves with the process by which vulnerabilities are identified, communicated, as well as the specifics of any particular vulnerability when it becomes known.
- The technology and cybersecurity controls to enable remote reprogramming of CIEDs are largely understood and available today. Before remote reprogramming can be implemented in clinical practice, health care providers, industry, regulatory agencies and patients will need to consider other factors to ensure health care delivery is safe and effective. These include which settings of the CIED should be remotely reprogrammable, boundaries within which the values of the parameters should be maintained, location of the patient when remote reprogramming is to be performed, and how to notify patients of reprogramming changes.

DISCLOSURE

Dr D.J. Slotwiner has received research support from Boston Scientific.

REFERENCES

1. Slotwiner D, Varma N, Akar JG, et al. HRS Expert Consensus Statement on Remote Interrogation and Monitoring for Cardiovascular Implantable Electronic Devices. Heart Rhythm: The Official Journal of the Heart Rhythm Society 12 (7): e69–100. DOI: doi: 10.1016/j.hrthm.2015.05.008.
2. Sanger DE, Perlroth N, Barnes JE. As understanding of Russian hacking grows, so does alarm. The New York Times 2021. Available at: https://www.nytimes.com/2021/01/02/us/politics/russian-hacking-government.html.
3. Green M. A few notes on MedSec and St. Jude medical 2018. Available at: https://blog.cryptographyengineering.com/2018/02/17/a-few-notes-on-medsec-and-st-jude-medical/. Accessed January 24, 2021.
4. How to avoid contactless card fraud [Internet]. Available at: https://www.equifax.co.uk/resources/identity-protection/how-to-avoid-contactless-card-fraud.html. Accessed January 23, 2021.
5. Ballard B. Only a tiny percentage of security vulnerabilities are actually exploited in the wild [Internet]. 2021. Available at: https://www.techradar.com/news/only-a-tiny-percentage-of-security-vulnerabilities-are-actually-exploited-in-the-wild. Accessed January 25, 2021.
6. Cimpanu C. Only 5.5% of all vulnerabilities are ever exploited in the wild [Internet] 2019. Available at: https://www.zdnet.com/article/only-5-5-of-all-vulnerabilities-are-ever-exploited-in-the-wild/. Accessed January 25, 2021.
7. Slotwiner DJ, Deering TF, Fu K, et al. Cybersecurity vulnerabilities of cardiac implantable electronic devices: communication strategies for clinicians—proceedings of the Heart Rhythm Society's Leadership Summit. Heart Rhythm 2018;15(7):e61–7.

Use of Smartphones and Wearables for Arrhythmia Monitoring

David J. Sanders, MD[a], Jeremiah Wasserlauf, MD, MS[a],
Rod S. Passman, MD, MSCE[b],*

KEYWORDS

• Arrhythmia • mhealth • Digital health • Atrial fibrillation

KEY POINTS

- Mobile health (mHealth), which uses patients' personal mobile wireless devices, can be used for ambulatory arrhythmia detection.
- Methods for arrhythmia detection can be classified as those that produce an electrocardiogram (ECG) tracing and those, such as photoplethysmography (PPG), that do not.
- Both ECG-based and PPG-based methods are accurate for atrial fibrillation (AF) detection. The role of these technologies for AF screening and quantification of AF burden is an area of active investigation.
- Routine use of mHealth for assessment of other arrhythmias and medical conditions, such as myocardial ischemia, are technically possible but require further study.
- Direct-to-consumer marketing can reach a wide range of patients but the data this generates may raise logistical and medical challenges.

Consumer smartphones and wearable devices now provide options for ambulatory rhythm monitoring that previously required medical-grade wearable or insertable cardiac monitors (ICMs). The role of mobile health (mHealth) has been studied perhaps most extensively for the diagnosis and management of atrial fibrillation (AF), but the applications are rapidly evolving to include other aspects of heart rhythm assessment and conditions across cardiology and medicine (Fig. 1). Expanding use of these devices raises several important questions about their accuracy, implications, and limitations. This review describes technical aspects of these devices, the current evidence base, and drawbacks and future directions.

A BRIEF HISTORY OF CARDIAC MONITORING: FROM MAIMONIDES TO INSERTABLE CARDIAC MONITORS

It was almost a millennium ago that Moses Maimonides first identified an irregular heartbeat.[1] The twelfth-century Spanish rabbi, philosopher, and physician wrote, "Any type of pulse with more than one irregularity is a direct result of an abnormal constitution [of humors] of which is also irregular,"[1] It can be speculated that he was referring to AF.[1,2]

In the intervening centuries, it was demonstrated that the heart's rhythmic beating was a consequence of coordinated electrical activity that could be recorded and studied. In 1887, in London, Augustus Waller became the first to trace

[a] Department of Internal Medicine, Division of Cardiology, Rush University, 1717 West Harrison Street, Suite 331, Chicago, IL 60612, USA; [b] Department of Internal Medicine, Division of Cardiology, Northwestern University Feinberg School of Medicine, 251 East Huron, Feinberg 8-503, Chicago, IL 60611, USA
* Corresponding author.
E-mail address: r-passman@northwestern.edu

Card Electrophysiol Clin 13 (2021) 509–522
https://doi.org/10.1016/j.ccep.2021.04.004

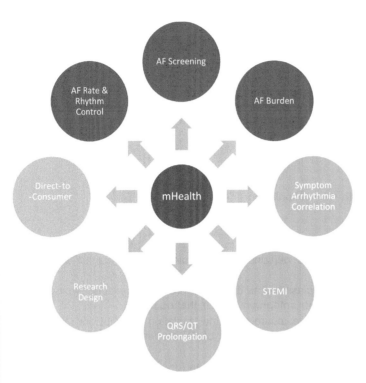

Fig. 1. Applications of mHealth to arrhythmia detection. mHealth has had an impact on diagnosis and management of a range of arrhythmias and its use likely will extend to more clinical scenarios. It also is reshaping cardiovascular care delivery and research design.

the heart's cyclic electrical changes, but his recordings were distorted and captured only 2 deflections.[3] Willem Einthoven, a Dutch physician working at the start of the twentieth century, expanded on Waller's work. Einthoven designed a string galvanometer that could produce clearer tracings and developed the standardized system of recording still used today.[3] For this work, which established the foundations of ECG, Einthoven was awarded the Nobel Prize in Physiology or Medicine in 1924.[3]

In the late 1940s, Norman "Jeff" Holter, working out of a laboratory in Helena, Montana, recognized the possibility of monitoring cardiac electrical activity outside of a clinical setting. He sought to develop a monitoring system that was portable and could record heart rhythms during patients' routine activities. His original device was a hulking 85-lb backpack with a long antenna that transmitted its electrocardiogram (ECG) signal by radio-frequency waves.[4] By the 1950s, Holter had achieved his goal of "radioelectrocardiology": he successfully miniaturized his device to a compact form and demonstrated tracings produced with adequate fidelity to detect pathology.[5]

The current arena of ambulatory ECG utilizes modern technology to capture the heart's electrical activity for extended durations in ambulatory settings.[6] Short-term external monitors, such as

the traditional Holter monitor or miniaturized patch monitors, offer full disclosure and event markers, but the relatively brief observation time limits diagnostic yield, especially for paroxysmal arrhythmias. ICMs extend observation time, and thus sensitivity, but are expensive, require an invasive procedure and vast infrastructure to adjudicate the stored data, and provide no real-time feedback to the patient.[7]

MOBILE HEALTH: AN OVERVIEW

mHealth is a form of health care delivery that utilizes patients' personal, mobile wireless communications devices. In its earliest form, mHealth focused on simple interventions, such as behavioral changes and education through text messaging.[8] The first use of consumer-grade heart monitors was in the training of competitive athletes in the 1970s. Over the past decade, devices have become increasingly sophisticated—built with accelerometers, cameras, and touch screens and powered by artificial intelligence.[8,9] This has enabled mHealth platforms to perform more complex diagnostics. Devices are capable of tracking an array of physiologic data—including a single-lead ECG and blood pressure—and transmitting them over wireless networks in real time.[9] Harnessing this power, there were more than

300,000 health care mobile applications available for use, with approximately 4 billion downloads as of 2017.[10]

Not only have mobile devices become "smart" but also their use is now ubiquitous. According to the Pew Research Center, in 2019, 96% of Americans owned some type of cellphone and 81% had a smartphone.[11] The widespread adoption of smart technology has made it possible for mHealth to reach a substantial number of people by directly marketing to consumers and incorporating health technology into the devices they already own. Barriers related to distance, cost, and time have the potential to be disrupted as the point of care is moved outside of traditional health care settings.[12] Mobile devices also may fill an important role in mitigating interruptions in care during the COVID-19 pandemic while reducing patient exposure to health care facilities.[13]

METHODS OF ARRHYTHMIA DETECTION

mHealth devices have been developed to assist in the management of several cardiac conditions, but their use may be studied most extensively for arrhythmia detection. There are several detection methods used to this end. These can be divided broadly into methods that do not produce an ECG—such as photoplethysmography (PPG)—and methods that produce an ECG tracing. Many devices employ a single arrhythmia detection method, although some, such as the Apple Watch, use a combination.

Photoplethysmography

PPG is a low-cost, noninvasive optical technique that measures changes in capillary blood volume.[14] A waveform is derived from the cyclic variation in absorbed light, a reflection of the changes in blood volume in the microvasculature with each heartbeat. These changes produce a high-frequency waveform that varies with the cardiac cycle and a low-frequency baseline influenced by respiration and autonomic tone.[15] PPG technology has been used in commercially available devices for the evaluation of a range of physiologic parameters, including oxygen saturation, blood pressure, and cardiac output, for more than a decade.[15]

More recently, utilizing light-emitting diodes (LEDs) and optical sensors already available on mHealth devices, PPG has been purposed to arrhythmia analysis. Smartphone users can direct the embedded light source onto their fingertip, and the phone's camera captures the reflected light. Similarly, smartwatches embedded with an LED light in the watch back can monitor a user's pulse continuously through the wrist. The PPG waveforms are analyzed by algorithms, programmed into the phone or watch, designed to distinguish AF from sinus rhythm by irregularity in the interval between pulsations.[16,17]

There are several PPG-based devices and applications that have been granted Food and Drug Administration (FDA) 510(k) clearance for AF detection[18,19] (**Table 1**). FibriCheck, developed by Qompium NV (Hasselt, Belgium), is an application that is downloaded onto a smartphone. It can be used with no additional equipment and is intended for intermittent rhythm checks. The Halo AF detection system (LIVMOR, Irvine, California), is a watch that performs rhythm analysis when the user is at rest or asleep. Both systems offer an interactive platform that allows users to engage with a health care professional if alerted to possible AF. Although there is growing interest in the use of PPG for screening of heart rhythm abnormalities, current guideline diagnostic criteria still require ECG confirmation.[20]

Photoplethysmography–based Algorithms for Atrial Fibrillation Detection

Although details of many signal processing methods are proprietary and therefore not published, the general computational approach to distinguishing sinus rhythm from AF exploits AF's irregular and random ventricular activation. For a given period of time, the PPG waveform is analyzed for variation in beat-to-beat intervals and morphology as well as the pattern's overall complexity and unpredictability.[17] Additionally, information extracted from the device's built-in accelerometer allows for filtering noise and motion artifact, which are major sources of error.[21]

Rhythm analysis relies on several statistical techniques, often employed in combination, including the root mean square of successive differences (RMSSD), Shannon entropy (ShE), Markov models, and Poincaré plot analysis (PPA).[17,21,22] RMSSD serves to quantify the RR interval variability, after normalizing for heart rate and is greater in patients with AF.[17] ShE and Markov Models are 2 different statistical approaches that compare segments of data for similarities and characterize the pattern's uncertainty.[17,23] PPA involves a geometric scatter diagram that examines the correlation between sequential data points over time and has been used to evaluate multiple physiologic systems.[24] When applied to rhythm assessment, analysis of the plot's shape has proved useful in discriminating AF from premature atrial contractions and premature ventricular contractions.[21,25]

Table 1
Devices for arrhythmia detection

Design/ Technique	Food and Drug Administration– cleared Devices	Clinical Applications	Advantages	Limitations
Smartphone PPG	FibriCheck	Single–time point AF detection	No additional hardware Interactive platform for medical care	Need ECG confirmation May miss short episodes Cannot be used for arrhythmias other than AF
Smartwatch PPG	LIVMOR Halo FibriCheck	AF detection	More likely to detect short AF episodes Passive AF evaluation during routine use Interactive platform for medical care	Need ECG confirmation Cannot be used for arrhythmias other than AF
Handheld ECG	KardiaMobile KardiaMobile 6L	Single–time point AF detection Postevent recorder for other arrhythmias	ECG tracing saved for physician review Potential to capture range of arrhythmias and ECG parameters Interactive platform for medical care/integration into EHR	Need additional hardware May miss short arrhythmic episodes
Smartwatch PPG and ECG	Apple Watch Samsung Galaxy Watch Fitbit Sense Verily Study Watch	AF detection	More likely to detect short AF episodes Passive AF evaluation during routine use Can confirm rhythm with ECG ECG could capture other arrhythmias	Monitoring not truly continuous—may underestimate or overestimate AF burden

Some signal processing algorithms assess the likelihood of AF by comparing results to thresholds established using explicit rules derived from validated databases.[23] These are simple enough that they can be programmed directly onto the device.[22] Although they generally have good diagnostic accuracy, they are challenged by atypical PPG user environments or in situations with poor signal quality, including circumstances, such as exercise, with high noise and motion artifact.[22,26–28]

Novel algorithms are powered by deep neural networks—a type of machine learning capable of producing increasingly nonlinear, abstract connections among data.[29] Convolutional neural networks, a subtype of deep learning, can assign weights and biases to each of their connections, and, because of their particularly high discriminatory capacity, frequently are used in medicine.[30] Deep learning algorithms are advantageous in their ability to learn new feature representations without explicit rules and may offer greater accuracy for a range of environments, especially those with noise.[23,26]

Electrocardiogram–based Methods for Arrhythmia Detection

With the addition of attachable external hardware, AliveCor (Mountain View, California) has developed an FDA 510(k) cleared personal ECG monitor, KardiaMobile, which provides a 30-second single-lead ECG using a smartphone.[31] The device consists of 2 battery-powered steel electrodes, which optionally can be secured to the back of a phone, on which users place their fingers. The captured signal is transmitted to the phone microphone by radiofrequency signal and then a tracing is displayed on the smartphone through the KardiaMobile application.

AliveCor's machine learning algorithm examines approximately 50 parameters from the generated tracing, including information regarding the RR intervals, morphology, and signal quality, and outputs whether or not the rhythm represents possible AF.[32] The tracing then can be stored and transmitted for physician review. Furthermore, because the KardiaMobile system is ECG-based, it has the potential to function as a postevent recorder and has been shown to be noninferior at detecting symptomatic arrhythmias compared with an external loop recorder.[33] The device has been used to record arrhythmias, including supraventricular tachycardia, ventricular tachycardia, and complete heart block.[34–36]

A newer iteration, KardiaMobile 6L, utilizes a third electrode placed on the left leg to generate a 6-lead ECG. This has the potential to facilitate the diagnosis of atrial flutter and provide additional information, such as ST segment changes, QT interval measurement, and morphologic assessment of arrhythmia complexes. Users of the AliveCor systems can purchase access to an interactive platform, which includes a cardiologist's review of the tracings and ability share tracings with caregivers.

Combination Electrocardiogram and Photoplethysmography Methods: Wrist-worn Wearables

A group of smartwatches has entered the realm of arrhythmia detection employing a combination of PPG-based and ECG-based methods. Together, these methods allow for passive monitoring for irregular rhythms and ECG confirmation. The Apple Watch, currently in its sixth iteration, is equipped with optical sensors embedded in the watch back, which use PPG to sample the user's heart rate every 2 hours to 4 hours. If heart rate irregularity is detected, the watch begins checking with greater frequency—as often as every 15 minutes. If 5 out of 6 consecutive samples over a 48-hour period are deemed irregular, the user is alerted to possible AF through the watch's "Irregular Rhythm Notification" feature.[37]

In addition to PPG analysis, the Apple Watch has ECG capability. The watch uses 1 electrode embedded in the crown and another in the watch back to record a single-lead ECG. The user applies a fingertip from the contralateral hand to the watch crown for 30 seconds. The tracing can be seen on the watch face or on a paired iPhone and then stored for future reference.[37] An advantage of watch-based rhythm analysis is that the PPG method can provide near-continuous rhythm assessment without requiring any action from the user, alongside ECG confirmation on demand.

Several other manufacturers have developed wrist-worn wearables that offer both passive PPG rhythm monitoring and single-lead ECG capability. Samsung, Fitbit, and Google's subsidiary Verily all have received FDA 510(k) clearance for AF detection applications—although the Verily device is not yet available to consumers.[38–40] Huawei's Honor Band has been studied for heart rhythm assessment and is commercially available

but does not have FDA clearance at the time of this writing.

Accuracy of Atrial Fibrillation Detection

Overall, PPG-based methods used for AF detection have been shown to be accurate in both smartphones and smartwatches. Multiple studies have found PPG algorithms capable of distinguishing sinus rhythm from AF with a sensitivity and specificity approaching or exceeding 95% compared with ECG.[17,21,41] A meta-analysis of 10 primary diagnostic accuracy studies using PPV signal acquired from a smartphone camera and applications across different manufacturers found sensitivity of 94.2% and specificity of 95.8%.[42]

PPG's application to real-world diagnostics was assessed in the Apple Heart Study. In the largest study of its kind, smartwatch-based PPG on the Apple Watch Series 1 or later was assessed for AF detection during routine use in a general population without preexisting AF.[43,44] It was a pragmatic, siteless, single-arm trial, which included more than 419,000 subjects monitored for AF with the Apple Watch.[43,44] Participants who received an irregular heart rhythm alert were sent a 7-day patch monitor for subsequent AF evaluation.[43,44]

Only 0.52% of all participants received an abnormal heart rhythm alert.[43] The low rate of irregular pulse notifications alleviates some concerns about false-positive detections that could occur in a healthy group of smartwatch users and reflects the young population included in the study, which had an average age of 41 years.[43] Irregular pulse notifications were sent to 3.1% of participants 65 years of age or older, and the average age of those who received an alert was 57 years.[43]

Of the patients who received an irregular rhythm alert, 20.8% returned the patch monitor for analysis, and AF was confirmed in 34% of cases.[43] This comparison may underestimate the positive predictive value of the algorithm given the time lag between the watch alert and wearing of the patch. For patients simultaneously wearing the Apple Watch and a patch monitor, possible AF alerts had an 84% positive predictive value. Enhancing yield ultimately may depend on targeting at-risk populations and optimizing the algorithm to detect brief AF episodes.[43]

The study's success at rapidly enrolling a large number of participants highlights the potential for virtual, pragmatic studies of consumer devices to scale more quickly and with fewer resources than traditional clinical trials.[43,45] Similar, prospective studies are ongoing. A trial to assess Fitbit's

PPG algorithm during typical use has completed enrollment with 450,000 participants and will compare the accuracy of its device to a single-lead patch monitor for the detection of AF.[46] This, and other studies, will need to validate the performance of the spectrum of PPG algorithms during typical use across a range of patient populations.

Handheld ECG-based systems also have demonstrated high diagnostic accuracy for AF compared with standard ECG or Holter monitor. For interpretable tracings, the AliveCor algorithm has been found highly accurate with sensitivity and specificity approaching or exceeding 95% in multiple studies.[32,47] The single-lead ECG has been shown to be interpretable by both cardiologists and primary care physicians.[47] One meta-analysis of 14 studies examining 7 different handheld devices found that physicians in both hospital and community settings can interpret the single-lead ECGs accurately compared with standard 12-lead ECGs or Holter monitors.[48]

Other Mobile Health Technologies for Arrhythmia Detection

Facial PPG (FPPG) applies the principles of PPG to facial video. The cyclic changes in capillary blood flow during the cardiac cycle result in subtle changes to facial color.[49] This can be captured by a standard digital video camera and the film analyzed for beat-to-beat variability consistent with AF.[49] In a prospective study of 217 patients, Yan and colleagues[50] showed that facial video from an iPhone camera analyzed using an FPPG-based application had 95% sensitivity and 96% specificity for distinguishing sinus rhythm and AF. As demonstrated in a proof-of-concept study, FPPG may present an opportunity for high throughput AF screening at a low cost.[51]

Mechanocardiography takes advantage of the microelectromechanical accelerometers and gyroscopes already embedded in the smartphone to detect the changes in cardiac motion with systole and diastole.[52] Then, similar to PPG, an algorithm evaluates the pattern of beat-to-beat intervals as well as the shape and randomness of the recorded signal to determine if a patient's rhythm is AF.[52] A small case-control study showed that the mechanocardiography algorithm distinguished AF from sinus rhythm with 95.3% sensitivity and 96% specificity.[53]

SCREENING FOR ATRIAL FIBRILLATION

AF is the most common heart rhythm disorder, affecting 33 million people worldwide.[54,55] In the United States, up to 9% of the population 65 years of age or older has AF, and the overall prevalence is projected to reach between 12.1 million and 15.9 million people by 2050.[56,57] Patients with AF are more likely to develop heart failure and dementia and have decreased quality of life.[20] Ischemic stroke is 5 times more likely in patients with AF, with larger infarct size and greater likelihood of death.[20,58] The economic impact of AF in the United States is estimated at $26 billion annually.[59] Despite this significant morbidity and the availability of effective oral anticoagulant therapy, the evidence to support widespread screening for AF, particularly with ECG, remains conflicting.

There are studies in which community-based AF screening has captured previously undetected AF at a considerable rate. In 1 study, single–time point checks with either ECG or palpation identified new AF in 1% of a general ambulatory population and in 1.4% of those older than 65.[60] The mSToPS trial randomized more than 2500 patients to receive a continuously worn patch monitor or usual care for 4 months.[61] AF was identified in 3.9% of patients who wore the patch compared with 0.9% of patients in the control arm.[61]

mHealth devices similarly may be an effective primary screening tool. In the REHEARSE-AF trial, more than 1000 patients aged 65 or older with a CHA_2DS_2-VASc score of at least 2 were randomized to receive either twice-weekly digital ECGs using KardiaMobile or routine care alone.[62] Over a 12-month period, patients in the study's experimental arm were significantly more likely to receive a new AF diagnosis, although the cost per AF diagnosis was $10,780, most of which was due to the cost of physician over-reads.[62] The DIGITAL-AF Study evaluated a PPG-based screening method: more than 12,000 enrolled participants were screened over a maximum period of 7 days and resulted in a cumulative diagnostic yield of 1.4%.[63]

To assess the effectiveness of single–time point screening a program with a single-lead ECG on a large scale, the VITAL-AF study randomized more than 35,000 patients aged 65 years or older to screening with the KardiaMobile device or usual care.[64] At 1 year, 1.52% of subjects in the screening group were diagnosed with new AF compared with 1.39% in the control group (relative risk 1.10; 95% CI, 0.92–1.30; $P = .30$).[64] Although this was a negative result for the overall study population, new AF diagnoses were significantly more frequent in the group of subjects aged 85 or over (4.05% vs 2.68%, respectively; $P = .02$).[64]

Long-term monitors, including ICMs, may overcome some of the limitations of single–time point rhythm assessments. They have increased sensitivity for AF detection and can quantify AF burden.[65,66] In patients with established risk factors for AF, ICMs detect a high prevalence of AF. The REVEAL AF, a multicenter study of patients without previously known AF but with elevated risk for AF and stroke, showed that ICMs detected AF in 40% of patients.[67] Similarly, the ASSERT-II investigators found that ICMs implanted in an older patient population without AF—but with risk factors for AF—detected subclinical AF at a rate of 34.4% per year.[65] Despite their high rate of AF detection and appropriateness in specific clinical scenarios, ICMs are not ideal as a general screening technology because of their cost, invasive implant procedure, and lack of real-time feedback to the patient.[68,69]

Near-continuous passive monitoring using smartwatch PPG may be more appropriate for AF screening. The feasibility of this type of model was demonstrated in a large-scale pragmatic study of more than 180,000 adults who underwent AF screening using 1 of several Huawei smart devices.[70] Although the population studied was young and yielded new AF at a rate of 0.23%, a positive alert led to engagement with an integrated AF management program in 95% of patients, and 80% of those with stroke risk were treated with anticoagulation.[70]

Smartwatch PPG also has been shown to be highly sensitive for detection of AF burden. A prior study by the authors' group assessed the accuracy of a smartwatch with a convolutional neural network algorithm for measurement of AF burden (proportion of time spent in AF), duration, and episodes in patients with paroxysmal AF compared with an ICM gold standard. Sensitivity exceeded 97% for all measures.[71]

Although assessment of AF burden in clinical practice and research settings has been limited by short durations of monitoring or the need for ICMs, mHealth devices now may enable more meaningful assessments of response to rhythm control strategies. In addition, as the relationship between AF burden and thrombotic complications increasingly is understood, mHealth devices also may permit more personalized prediction of AF complications, such as stroke.[72]

Although the initial research on AF screening has been promising, no studies, as yet, have examined how an mHealth screening program might have an impact on hard outcomes. The ongoing Heartline hopes to enroll 150,000 patients 65 years or older to assess if an AF screening program with the Apple Watch Series 5 results in earlier AF detection, earlier direct oral anticoagulation prescriptions, or differences in clinical outcomes, such as death, stroke, and myocardial infarction.[73]

Screening targeted at older patients and those with specific risk factors might be most effective and more likely to result in intervention.[74,75] Patients with cryptogenic stroke previously have been demonstrated to have up to 30% prevalence of occult AF when screened using an ICM.[76] Multiple professional society guidelines recommend ambulatory cardiac monitoring for AF after stroke.[77,78] The role of mHealth to monitor these patients for occult AF requires further study and also must address the impact of interruptions to monitoring that occur during device battery charging.[71]

Although mHealth may serve as an effective tool to screen for subclinical AF, studies still are needed to characterize the potential benefits of anticoagulation for device-detected AF, including by mHealth devices. Although current guidelines recommend anticoagulant therapy on the basis of CHA_2DS_2-VASc score irrespective of AF pattern, patients with subclinical AF detected on devices were not included in studies of anticoagulant therapy. Increased duration and burden of AF are associated with increased risk for arterial embolic events at durations of 24 hours or less. There is no consensus on a single threshold that merits anticoagulation or other treatment. Very short episodes may not require action beyond continued monitoring.[79–81] Combining CHA_2DS_2-VASc score with AF characteristics, such as burden and duration, may refine risk prediction further.[82] Although personalizing stroke risk prediction in this way traditionally has been impractical, mHealth devices may fulfill an important need for long-term information on AF characteristics previously off-limits to clinical and research settings without an implanted cardiac device.

MOBILE HEALTH IN MANAGEMENT OF ESTABLISHED ATRIAL FIBRILLATION

Beyond initial AF diagnosis, mHealth has potential applicability to patients with established AF in several ways. Given the high proportion of asymptomatic AF, mHealth could serve to assess the efficacy of rhythm-control interventions, including antiarrhythmic medications and ablation.[83] It also can be used to assess the toxicity of antiarrhythmic drugs that produce increases in QRS or QT intervals. Guidelines use a 30-second threshold to define postablation AF recurrence.[84] Use of this binary endpoint may obscure meaningful reductions in AF burden than can be captured only with extended continuous monitoring.[85] Similarly, patients treated with a rate-control approach could be monitored for adequate control of their heart rate in AF.[86] Smartphone-based interventions to assess for AF recurrence and motivational texting to improve AF-based quality of life are ongoing.[87]

EXERCISE AND ATRIAL FIBRILLATION

The relationship between exercise and AF is incompletely understood. Prior studies have shown that aerobic interval training can reduce AF burden and symptoms as well as improve quality of life.[88] By contrast, high-intensity and endurance physical activity have been associated with an increased incidence of AF.[89] Current professional society guidelines recommend 150 minutes of moderate intensity physical activity per week; however, the optimal duration and intensity of exercise to benefit patients with AF have not been established.[90] mHealth devices, which can obtain an array of data on physical activity in addition to heart rate and rhythm assessment, may have a role in clarifying this relationship.

MOBILE HEALTH AND OBSTRUCTIVE SLEEP APNEA

Obstructive sleep apnea (OSA) is a form of sleep-disordered breathing with an estimated global prevalence of nearly 1 billion people.[91] OSA is common in patients with AF and can promote anatomic and electrical atrial remodeling, which serves as a substrate for AF.[92] OSA treatment with continuous positive airway pressure therapy reduces risk of AF recurrence after cardioversion or catheter ablation.[93] Early diagnosis and treatment in these patients would be beneficial. The standard for OSA diagnosis is in-laboratory polysomnography, although home portable monitors, such as wrist actigraphy, can be used as adjuncts.[94] An algorithm for a wireless patch monitor was demonstrated to determine the apnea-hypopnea index with accuracy comparable to polysomnography.[95] Future research is necessary to understand the role of consumer mHealth devices further in diagnosis and management of OSA in the home environment or the potential for their use in titrating and monitoring response to OSA therapies.

MOBILE HEALTH AND OTHER ARRHYTHMIAS AND ELECTROCARDIOGRAPHIC PARAMETERS

There is significant potential to expand the use of mHealth devices to heart rhythm applications beyond AF. ECG-based mHealth devices can be used to capture and store tracings for clinician review and do not necessarily need an algorithm's analysis to be impactful. Two case reports describe patients with syncope who obtained tracings from their mHealth devices—one with KardiaMobile and the other with Apple Watch—during symptoms and each identified ventricular tachycardia, allowing physicians to direct appropriate care.[35,96]

PPG-based methods will require advanced algorithms to detect differences among rhythms. The PULSE-SMART study showed that a novel algorithm using pulse wave signals obtained from an iPhone reliably could distinguish among sinus rhythm, AF, premature atrial contractions, and premature ventricular contractions.[22]

As discussed previously, in the role of symptom-arrhythmia correlation, current ECG-based mHealth devices have the ability to function as post-event recorders—that is, a tracing or analysis can be obtained after the patient notices their symptoms, but true continuous monitoring and full disclosure are not possible. One of the most important features of ambulatory cardiac monitoring is identification of arrhythmia at the time of symptoms. This limits identification of symptoms that are very short-lived or those, such as syncope, that fully incapacitate the patient. This type of monitoring still may provide a benefit under some circumstances. In a prospective randomized trial, 243 patients presenting to an emergency department with symptoms of palpitations or presyncope were more likely to have their symptomatic rhythm identified and to have quicker identification if given an AliveCor mobile ECG device than usual care.[97] The results of this study do suggest that mHealth devices still may be useful if able to capture a rhythm during a prodromal period or immediately after an event.

As ECG-based mHealth systems become more directly comparable to a 12-lead ECG, broader applications that require precise evaluation of ECG parameters may become possible. ECG-based mHealth systems have the potential to serve as an alternative to inpatient observation for initiation of antiarrhythmic drugs, including dofetilide and sotalol, which have QT interval–prolonging potential and an associated risk of torsades de pointes. Two small studies showed comparable accuracy to lead I or II on a 12-lead ECG for determining the corrected QT interval in patients in sinus rhythm beginning treatment with oral QT-prolonging antiarrhythmic drugs.[98,99] This has clinical applicability to the use of other QT-prolonging medications, such as hydroxychloroquine and azithromycin, that were proposed for use early in the worldwide experience with COVID-19 infection.[100]

Timely diagnosis and management of ST-segment elevation myocardial infarction (STEMI) are critical because delays are associated with increased morbidity and mortality.[101] An ICM equipped with a system to alert patients to an evolving STEMI has been shown to reduce the time from detection to arrival at a medical facility.[102] ECG-based mHealth systems capable of analyzing a patient's ST segment could aid in reducing time to presentation. As a proof of concept, 1 study showed that patients could reliably use a noninvasive device to self-record 3-lead ECGs, making the diagnosis of STEMI.[103] In a case report, it now has been shown that the Apple Watch Series 4 is capable of generating a 3-lead ECG and diagnosing STEMI.[104] Further research is necessary to determine diagnostic accuracy, patient usability, effect on total ischemic time, and outcomes in larger cohorts.

A SHIFT IN CLINICAL PRACTICE: THE CHALLENGES AHEAD

The rapid development and use of mHealth devices for cardiac evaluation represent a paradigm shift in health care delivery. Many of these digital devices are marketed and sold directly to consumers, often bypassing a traditional pathway of research and expert evaluation prior to individual patient use.[105] This model offers an opportunity to reach a wide range of patients, encourages patient engagement, and empowers patients to take control of their own health care.[106]

The change extends to research design and implementation. As exemplified by the Apple Heart Study, mHealth facilitates large-scale real-world study design with virtual assessments. By bypassing traditional geographic and temporal constraints, broad and rapid study enrollment is possible at a reduced cost per patient.[45] But these designs may face challenges due to their dependence on subject engagement and accurate self-reporting.[45]

The direct distribution of medical devices to consumers also introduces several challenges. Devices may reach the marketplace before scientific evaluation has established what constitutes an appropriate use. Patients, who can purchase devices without consulting a doctor, may confront difficulty distinguishing between clinically tested and untested equipment. Furthermore, because many clinical situations have not been studied, the physician may be tasked to make treatment decisions on device obtained data without clear guidance.

Beyond the implications for medical decision making, mHealth's use in health care delivery raises several logistical, legal, and ethical challenges. Wearable devices accumulate a vast amount of data and have the potential to overload both physicians and consumers.[9] Systems need to be implemented to effectively distill the information that is most clinically useful.[9] Physician responsibility to oversee this data still is uncertain. Integrating results into the electronic health record (EHR) poses another challenge. AliveCor has created a platform that allows physicians to incorporate data into the records, along with Current Procedural Terminology codes, which offers an opportunity for reimbursement.[107] This type of integration, however, is inconsistent across platforms. Finally, the law regarding patient privacy and malpractice liability is not fully established. Patient data may not be protected when obtained using applications outside of the health care setting.[108] Physician liability also is uncertain, but claims against physicians likely would depend on an accepted standard of care using mHealth and an established physician-patient relationship.[108]

There is excitement about the possibility that mHealth could reach people who otherwise might be left out by the health care system, especially because smartphone ownership still is high among those of lower socioeconomic status.[11] But it also is possible that mHealth could exacerbate disparities. In particular, older patients, who may benefit most from health care interventions, may be the least likely to own a smart device or have facility with their use.[11,109]

SUMMARY

The emergence of mHealth presents an opportunity for noninvasive ambulatory cardiac monitoring in a range of patients without the cost and constraints of traditional medical-grade monitors. mHealth may have greatest impact in the diagnosis and management of AF, alongside artificial intelligence–driven rhythm analysis. Clinical applications for arrhythmia management are growing with implications for patient engagement, point-of-care management, and research design. As mHealth devices become fixtures in medical practice, clarification in health policy will be needed to address the potential of increased burden of patient data and liability for health care providers. Future efforts from mHealth developers will need to focus on tabulation of data from multiple modalities in a way that can be analyzed easily, submitted for reimbursement, and integrated with the EHR.

CLINICS CARE POINTS

- mHealth devices are becoming increasingly common and generate an array of health data, including ECG tracings.
- ECG-based recordings are advantageous in that they satisfy a gold standard for AF diagnosis by a clinician. PPG has the potential to offer continuous monitoring for AF as well as quantification of AF burden.
- Algorithms for AF detection have been shown to be accurate compared with standard diagnostic modalities, but their precise clinical applications still are being determined.
- mHealth devices could represent an alternative to medical-grade equipment for AF screening, evaluation of the QT interval, and monitoring patients on antiarrhythmic medications. The COVID-19 pandemic has accelerated adoption of these devices by some clinicians to enable clinical care outside of traditional health care settings.
- mHealth can improve patient engagement and generate a wealth of health care data. Key questions remain in regard to optimal integration of this data with EHRs and management of data overload as well as responsibility and liability for information obtained.

DISCLOSURES

Rod S. Passman, MD, MSCE: Johnson and Johnson (advisory board), Medtronic (advisory boards), and UpToDate (royalties); Jeremiah Wasserlauf, MD, MS: Stryker (consulting) and Sanofi (consulting/speaking); and David J. Sanders, MD: none.

REFERENCES

1. Rosner F. Moses Maimonides and diseases of the chest. Chest 1971;60(1):68–72.
2. Luscher TF. Atrial fibrillation and arrhythmias: novel risk assessment, proper anticoagulation, and ablation. Eur Heart J 2018;39(16):1317–21.
3. Barold SS. Willem Einthoven and the birth of clinical electrocardiography a hundred years ago. Card Electrophysiol Rev 2003;7(1):99–104.
4. Barold SS, Norman J. "Jeff" Holter-"Father" of ambulatory ECG monitoring. J Interv Card Electrophysiol 2005;14(2):117–8.
5. Holter NJ. Radioelectrocardiography: a new technique for cardiovascular studies. Ann N Y Acad Sci 1957;65(6):913–23.
6. Steinberg JS, Varma N, Cygankiewicz I, et al. 2017 ISHNE-HRS expert consensus statement on ambulatory ECG and external cardiac monitoring/telemetry. Ann Noninvasive Electrocardiol 2017;22(3):e55–96.
7. Lee R, Mittal S. Utility and limitations of long-term monitoring of atrial fibrillation using an implantable loop recorder. Heart Rhythm 2018;15(2):287–95.
8. Turakhia MP, Kaiser DW. Transforming the care of atrial fibrillation with mobile health. J Interv Card Electrophysiol 2016;47(1):45–50.
9. Steinhubl SR, Muse ED, Topol EJ. The emerging field of mobile health. Sci Transl Med 2015;7(283):283rv3.
10. Mahmood A, Kedia S, Wyant DK, et al. Use of mobile health applications for health-promoting behavior among individuals with chronic medical conditions. Digit Health 2019;5. 2055207619882181.
11. Mobile Fact sheet [Website]. Pew Research Center; 2019. Available at: https://www.pewresearch.org/internet/fact-sheet/mobile/.
12. Silva BM, Rodrigues JJ, de la Torre Diez I, et al. Mobile-health: a review of current state in 2015. J Biomed Inform 2015;56:265–72.
13. Services USDoHaH. Enforcement policy for non-invasive Remote monitoring devices used to support patient monitoring during the coronavirus disease 2019 (COVID-19) public health emergency. Guidance fo Industry and Food Drug Administration Staff; 2020. p. 12. Available at: https://www.fda.gov/regulatory-information/search-fda-guidance-documents/enforcement-policy-non-invasive-remote-monitoring-devices-used-support-patient-monitoring-during.
14. Castaneda D, Esparza A, Ghamari M, et al. A review on wearable photoplethysmography sensors and their potential future applications in health care. Int J Biosens Bioelectron 2018;4(4):195–202.
15. Allen J. Photoplethysmography and its application in clinical physiological measurement. Physiol Meas 2007;28(3):R1–39.
16. Conroy T, Guzman JH, Hall B, et al. Detection of atrial fibrillation using an earlobe photoplethysmographic sensor. Physiol Meas 2017;38(10):1906–18.
17. McManus DD, Lee J, Maitas O, et al. A novel application for the detection of an irregular pulse using an iPhone 4S in patients with atrial fibrillation. Heart Rhythm 2013;10(3):315–9.
18. Browning SC. Premarket notification for LIVMOR HALO AF detection system (K201208). Administration USFD; 2020. Available at: https://www.accessdata.fda.gov/cdrh_docs/pdf20/K201208.pdf.
19. Drummond A. Premarket notification for FibriCheck (K173872). Administration USFD; 2018. Available

at: https://www.accessdata.fda.gov/cdrh_docs/pdf17/K173872.pdf.

20. January CT, Wann LS, Alpert JS, et al. 2014 AHA/ACC/HRS guideline for the management of patients with atrial fibrillation: executive summary: a report of the American College of Cardiology/American Heart Association Task Force on practice guidelines and the Heart Rhythm Society. Circulation 2014;130(23):2071–104.

21. Bashar SK, Han D, Hajeb-Mohammadalipour S, et al. Atrial fibrillation detection from wrist photoplethysmography signals using smartwatches. Sci Rep 2019;9(1):15054.

22. Mc MD, Chong JW, Soni A, et al. PULSE-SMART: pulse-based arrhythmia discrimination using a novel smartphone application. J Cardiovasc Electrophysiol 2016;27(1):51–7.

23. Pereira T, Tran N, Gadhoumi K, et al. Photoplethysmography based atrial fibrillation detection: a review. NPJ Digit Med 2020;3:3.

24. Satti R, Abid NU, Bottaro M, et al. The application of the extended Poincare plot in the analysis of physiological variabilities. Front Physiol 2019;10:116.

25. Bashar SK, Han D, Zieneddin F, et al. Preliminary results on Density Poincare plot based atrial fibrillation detection from premature atrial/ventricular contractions(.). Annu Int Conf IEEE Eng Med Biol Soc 2020;2020:2594–7.

26. Torres-Soto J, Ashley EA. Multi-task deep learning for cardiac rhythm detection in wearable devices. NPJ Digit Med 2020;3:116.

27. Elgendi M. Optimal signal quality index for photoplethysmogram signals. Bioengineering (Basel). 2016;3(4):21.

28. Zhang Z, Pi Z, Liu B. TROIKA: a general framework for heart rate monitoring using wrist-type photoplethysmographic signals during intensive physical exercise. IEEE Trans Biomed Eng 2015;62(2):522–31.

29. LeCun Y, Bengio Y, Hinton G. Deep learning. Nature 2015;521(7553):436–44.

30. Johnson KW, Torres Soto J, Glicksberg BS, et al. Artificial intelligence in cardiology. J Am Coll Cardiol 2018;71(23):2668–79.

31. Zuckerman BD. 510(k) premarket notification for KardiaMobile (K140933) 2014. Available at: https://www.accessdata.fda.gov/cdrh_docs/pdf14/K140933.pdf.

32. William AD, Kanbour M, Callahan T, et al. Assessing the accuracy of an automated atrial fibrillation detection algorithm using smartphone technology: the iREAD Study. Heart Rhythm 2018;15(10):1561–5.

33. Narasimha D, Hanna N, Beck H, et al. Validation of a smartphone-based event recorder for arrhythmia detection. Pacing Clin Electrophysiol 2018;41(5):487–94.

34. Tabing A, Harrell TE, Romero S, et al. Supraventricular tachycardia diagnosed by smartphone ECG. BMJ Case Rep 2017;2017. https://doi.org/10.1136/bcr-2016-217197.

35. Waks JW, Fein AS, Das S. Wide complex tachycardia recorded with a smartphone cardiac rhythm monitor. JAMA Intern Med 2015;175(3):437–9.

36. Nyotowidjojo I, Erickson RP, Lee KS. Crowd-sourcing syncope diagnosis: mobile smartphone ECG apps. Am J Med 2016;129(4):e17–8.

37. Using Apple watch for arrhythmia detection. In: White Paper. Apple Incorporated; 2020.

38. Paulsen JE. 510(k) premarket notification for samsung ECG monitor application (K201168) 2020. Available at: https://www.accessdata.fda.gov/cdrh_docs/pdf20/K201168.pdf.

39. Paulsen JE. 510(k) premarket notification for Fitbit ECG App (K200948) 2020. Available at: https://www.accessdata.fda.gov/cdrh_docs/pdf20/K200948.pdf.

40. Shih J. 510(k) premarket notification for study watch with irregular pulse monitor (K192415) 2020. Available at: https://www.accessdata.fda.gov/cdrh_docs/pdf19/K192415.pdf.

41. Krivoshei L, Weber S, Burkard T, et al. Smart detection of atrial fibrillationdagger. Europace 2017;19(5):753–7.

42. O'Sullivan JW, Grigg S, Crawford W, et al. Accuracy of smartphone camera applications for detecting atrial fibrillation: a systematic review and meta-analysis. JAMA Netw Open 2020;3(4):e202064.

43. Perez MV, Mahaffey KW, Hedlin H, et al. Large-scale assessment of a smartwatch to identify atrial fibrillation. N Engl J Med 2019;381(20):1909–17.

44. Turakhia MP, Desai M, Hedlin H, et al. Rationale and design of a large-scale, app-based study to identify cardiac arrhythmias using a smartwatch: the Apple Heart Study. Am Heart J 2019;207:66–75.

45. Tarakji KG, Silva J, Chen LY, et al. Digital health and the care of the patient with arrhythmia: what every electrophysiologist needs to Know. Circ Arrhythm Electrophysiol 2020;13(11):e007953.

46. Validation of software for assessment of atrial fibrillation from PPG data acquired by a wearable smartwatch ClinicalTrials.gov. U.S. National Library of Medicine; 2021. Available at: https://clinicaltrials.gov/ct2/show/NCT04380415.

47. Koshy AN, Sajeev JK, Negishi K, et al. Accuracy of blinded clinician interpretation of single-lead smartphone electrocardiograms and a proposed clinical workflow. Am Heart J 2018;205:149–53.

48. Wong KC, Klimis H, Lowres N, et al. Diagnostic accuracy of handheld electrocardiogram devices in detecting atrial fibrillation in adults in community versus hospital settings: a systematic review and meta-analysis. Heart 2020;106(16):1211–7.

49. Couderc JP, Kyal S, Mestha LK, et al. Detection of atrial fibrillation using contactless facial video monitoring. Heart Rhythm 2015;12(1):195–201.

50. Yan BP, Lai WHS, Chan CKY, et al. Contact-free screening of atrial fibrillation by a smartphone using facial pulsatile photoplethysmographic signals. J Am Heart Assoc 2018;7(8):e008585.

51. Yan BP, Lai WHS, Chan CKY, et al. High-throughput, contact-free detection of atrial fibrillation from video with deep learning. JAMA Cardiol 2020;5(1):105–7.

52. Lahdenoja O, Hurnanen T, Iftikhar Z, et al. Atrial fibrillation detection via accelerometer and gyroscope of a smartphone. IEEE J Biomed Health Inform 2018;22(1):108–18.

53. Jaakkola J, Jaakkola S, Lahdenoja O, et al. Mobile phone detection of atrial fibrillation with mechanocardiography: the MODE-AF study (mobile phone detection of atrial fibrillation). Circulation 2018; 137(14):1524–7.

54. Rahman F, Kwan GF, Benjamin EJ. Global epidemiology of atrial fibrillation. Nat Rev Cardiol 2014; 11(11):639–54.

55. Chugh SS, Havmoeller R, Narayanan K, et al. Worldwide epidemiology of atrial fibrillation: a global burden of disease 2010 study. Circulation 2014;129(8):837–47.

56. McManus DD, Rienstra M, Benjamin EJ. An update on the prognosis of patients with atrial fibrillation. Circulation 2012;126(10):e143–6.

57. Miyasaka Y, Barnes ME, Gersh BJ, et al. Secular trends in incidence of atrial fibrillation in Olmsted County, Minnesota, 1980 to 2000, and implications on the projections for future prevalence. Circulation 2006;114(2):119–25.

58. Saxena R, Lewis S, Berge E, et al. Risk of early death and recurrent stroke and effect of heparin in 3169 patients with acute ischemic stroke and atrial fibrillation in the International Stroke Trial. Stroke 2001;32(10):2333–7.

59. Kim MH, Johnston SS, Chu BC, et al. Estimation of total incremental health care costs in patients with atrial fibrillation in the United States. Circ Cardiovasc Qual Outcomes 2011;4(3):313–20.

60. Lowres N, Neubeck L, Redfern J, et al. Screening to identify unknown atrial fibrillation. A systematic review. Thromb Haemost 2013;110(2):213–22.

61. Steinhubl SR, Waalen J, Edwards AM, et al. Effect of a home-based wearable continuous ECG monitoring patch on detection of undiagnosed atrial fibrillation: the mSToPS randomized clinical trial. JAMA 2018;320(2):146–55.

62. Halcox JPJ, Wareham K, Cardew A, et al. Assessment of remote heart rhythm sampling using the AliveCor heart monitor to screen for atrial fibrillation: the REHEARSE-AF study. Circulation 2017; 136(19):1784–94.

63. Verbrugge FH, Nuyens D, Vandervoort PM. Mass screening for AF with only the Use of a smartphone: the DIGITAL-AF trial: American college of cardiology 2018. Available at: https://www.acc.org/latest-in-cardiology/articles/2018/12/04/08/26/mass-screening-for-af-with-only-the-use-of-a-smartphone.

64. Lubitz SA, Atlas S, Ashburner JM, et al. Abstract 18676: Screening for atrial fibrillation in older adults at primary care visits using single lead electrocardiograms: the VITAL-AF study. The American Heart Association Scientific Sessions: CIRCULATION; 2020. https://doi.org/10.1161/CIR.0000000000000940.

65. Healey JS, Alings M, Ha A, et al. Subclinical atrial fibrillation in older patients. Circulation 2017; 136(14):1276–83.

66. Sanna T, Diener HC, Passman RS, et al. Cryptogenic stroke and underlying atrial fibrillation. N Engl J Med 2014;370(26):2478–86.

67. Reiffel JA, Verma A, Kowey PR, et al. Incidence of previously undiagnosed atrial fibrillation using insertable cardiac monitors in a high-risk population: the REVEAL AF study. JAMA Cardiol 2017;2(10): 1120–7.

68. Tomson TT, Passman R. Current and emerging uses of insertable cardiac monitors: evaluation of syncope and monitoring for atrial fibrillation. Cardiol Rev 2017;25(1):22–9.

69. Silveira I, Sousa MJ, Antunes N, et al. Efficacy and safety of implantable loop recorder: experience of A center. J Atr Fibrillation 2016;9(2):1425.

70. Guo Y, Wang H, Zhang H, et al. Mobile photoplethysmographic technology to detect atrial fibrillation. J Am Coll Cardiol 2019;74(19):2365–75.

71. Wasserlauf J, You C, Patel R, et al. Smartwatch performance for the detection and quantification of atrial fibrillation. Circ Arrhythm Electrophysiol 2019;12(6):e006834.

72. Go AS, Reynolds K, Yang J, et al. Association of burden of atrial fibrillation with risk of ischemic stroke in adults with paroxysmal atrial fibrillation: the KP-rhythm study. JAMA Cardiol 2018;3(7):601–8.

73. A study to investigate if early atrial fibrillation (AF) diagnosis reduces risk of events like stroke in the real-world ClinicalTrials.gov. U.S. National Library of Medicine; 2020. Available at: https://clinicaltrials.gov/ct2/show/NCT04276441.

74. Freedman B, Camm J, Calkins H, et al. Screening for atrial fibrillation: a report of the AF-SCREEN international collaboration. Circulation 2017;135(19): 1851–67.

75. Svennberg E, Engdahl J, Al-Khalili F, et al. Mass screening for untreated atrial fibrillation: the STROKESTOP study. Circulation 2015;131(25):2176–84.

76. Sanna T, Diener HC, Passman RS, et al. Cryptogenic stroke and atrial fibrillation. N Engl J Med 2014;371(13):1261.

77. Schnabel RB, Haeusler KG, Healey JS, et al. Searching for atrial fibrillation poststroke: a white paper of the AF-SCREEN international collaboration. Circulation 2019;140(22):1834–50.

78. Kirchhof P, Benussi S, Kotecha D, et al. 2016 ESC guidelines for the management of atrial fibrillation developed in collaboration with EACTS. Rev Esp Cardiol (Engl Ed) 2017;70(1):50.

79. Glotzer TV, Hellkamp AS, Zimmerman J, et al. Atrial high rate episodes detected by pacemaker diagnostics predict death and stroke: report of the Atrial Diagnostics Ancillary Study of the MOde Selection Trial (MOST). Circulation 2003;107(12):1614–9.

80. Healey JS, Connolly SJ, Gold MR, et al. Subclinical atrial fibrillation and the risk of stroke. N Engl J Med 2012;366(2):120–9.

81. Glotzer TV, Daoud EG, Wyse DG, et al. The relationship between daily atrial tachyarrhythmia burden from implantable device diagnostics and stroke risk: the TRENDS study. Circ Arrhythm Electrophysiol 2009;2(5):474–80.

82. Kaplan RM, Koehler J, Ziegler PD, et al. Stroke risk as a function of atrial fibrillation duration and CHA2DS2-VASc score. Circulation 2019;140(20):1639–46.

83. Passman RS. Monitoring for AF: identifying the burden of atrial fibrillation and assessing post-ablation. J Innov Card Rhythm Manag 2017;8(1):2575–82.

84. Calkins H, Hindricks G, Cappato R, et al. 2017 HRS/EHRA/ECAS/APHRS/SOLAECE expert consensus statement on catheter and surgical ablation of atrial fibrillation. Europace 2018;20(1):e1–160.

85. Andrade JG, Champagne J, Dubuc M, et al. Cryoballoon or radiofrequency ablation for atrial fibrillation assessed by continuous monitoring: a randomized clinical trial. Circulation 2019;140(22):1779–88.

86. Koshy AN, Sajeev JK, Nerlekar N, et al. Smart watches for heart rate assessment in atrial arrhythmias. Int J Cardiol 2018;266:124–7.

87. Caceres BA, Hickey KT, Bakken SB, et al. Mobile electrocardiogram monitoring and health-related quality of life in patients with atrial fibrillation: findings from the iPhone Helping evaluate atrial fibrillation rhythm through technology (iHEART) study. J Cardiovasc Nurs 2020;35(4):327–36.

88. Malmo V, Nes BM, Amundsen BH, et al. Aerobic interval training reduces the burden of atrial fibrillation in the short term: a randomized trial. Circulation 2016;133(5):466–73.

89. Aizer A, Gaziano JM, Cook NR, et al. Relation of vigorous exercise to risk of atrial fibrillation. Am J Cardiol 2009;103(11):1572–7.

90. Piercy KI, Troiano RP. Physical activity guidelines for Americans from the US department of health and human services. Circ Cardiovasc Qual Outcomes 2018;11(11):e005263.

91. Benjafield AV, Ayas NT, Eastwood PR, et al. Estimation of the global prevalence and burden of obstructive sleep apnoea: a literature-based analysis. Lancet Respir Med 2019;7(8):687–98.

92. Anter E, Di Biase L, Contreras-Valdes FM, et al. Atrial substrate and triggers of paroxysmal atrial fibrillation in patients with obstructive sleep apnea. Circ Arrhythm Electrophysiol 2017;10(11):e005407.

93. Qureshi WT, Nasir UB, Alqalyoobi S, et al. Meta-analysis of continuous positive airway pressure as a therapy of atrial fibrillation in obstructive sleep apnea. Am J Cardiol 2015;116(11):1767–73.

94. Epstein LJ, Kristo D, Strollo PJ Jr, et al. Clinical guideline for the evaluation, management and long-term care of obstructive sleep apnea in adults. J Clin Sleep Med 2009;5(3):263–76.

95. Selvaraj N, Narasimhan R. Automated prediction of the apnea-hypopnea index using a wireless patch sensor. Annu Int Conf IEEE Eng Med Biol Soc 2014;2014:1897–900.

96. Ringwald M, Crich A, Beysard N. Smart watch recording of ventricular tachycardia: case study. Am J Emerg Med 2020;38(4):849. e3-5.

97. Reed MJ, Grubb NR, Lang CC, et al. Multi-centre randomised controlled trial of a smartphone-based event recorder alongside standard care versus standard care for patients presenting to the emergency department with palpitations and pre-syncope: the IPED (investigation of palpitations in the ED) study. EClinicalMedicine 2019;8:37–46.

98. Chung EH, Guise KD. QTC intervals can be assessed with the AliveCor heart monitor in patients on dofetilide for atrial fibrillation. J Electrocardiol 2015;48(1):8–9.

99. Garabelli P, Stavrakis S, Albert M, et al. Comparison of QT interval readings in normal sinus rhythm between a smartphone heart monitor and a 12-lead ECG for healthy volunteers and inpatients receiving sotalol or dofetilide. J Cardiovasc Electrophysiol 2016;27(7):827–32.

100. Giudicessi JR, Noseworthy PA, Friedman PA, et al. Urgent guidance for navigating and circumventing the QTc-prolonging and torsadogenic potential of possible pharmacotherapies for coronavirus disease 19 (COVID-19). Mayo Clin Proc 2020;95(6):1213–21.

101. Scholz KH, Maier SKG, Maier LS, et al. Impact of treatment delay on mortality in ST-segment elevation myocardial infarction (STEMI) patients presenting with and without haemodynamic instability: results from the German prospective, multicentre FITT-STEMI trial. Eur Heart J 2018;39(13):1065–74.

102. Gibson CM, Holmes D, Mikdadi G, et al. Implantable cardiac alert system for early recognition of ST-segment elevation myocardial infarction. J Am Coll Cardiol 2019;73(15):1919–27.

103. Van Heuverswyn F, De Buyzere M, Coeman M, et al. Feasibility and performance of a device for automatic self-detection of symptomatic acute coronary artery occlusion in outpatients with coronary artery disease: a multicentre observational study. Lancet Digit Health 2019; 1(2):e90–9.

104. Avila CO. Novel use of Apple watch 4 to obtain 3-lead electrocardiogram and detect cardiac ischemia. Perm J 2019;23.

105. Ding EY, Marcus GM, McManus DD. Emerging technologies for identifying atrial fibrillation. Circ Res 2020;127(1):128–42.

106. Topol E. Digital medicine: empowering both patients and clinicians. Lancet 2016;388(10046): 740–1.

107. A guide to remote patient monitoring. AliveCor, Incoporated; 2019. Available at: https://clinicians. alivecor.com/documents/AliveCor%20Remote% 20Patient%20Monitoring%20Guide.pdf.

108. Yang YT, Silverman RD. Mobile health applications: the patchwork of legal and liability issues suggests strategies to improve oversight. Health Aff (Millwood) 2014;33(2):222–7.

109. Neubeck L, Lowres N, Benjamin EJ, et al. The mobile revolution–using smartphone apps to prevent cardiovascular disease. Nat Rev Cardiol 2015; 12(6):350–60.

Remote Monitoring of the QT Interval and Emerging Indications for Arrhythmia Prevention

Silvia Castelletti, MD[a], Bo Gregers Winkel, MD, PhD[b], Peter J. Schwartz, MD[a,*]

KEYWORDS

- Long QT syndrome • Idiopathic ventricular fibrillation • Remote QT interval monitoring
- Cardiac arrhythmias • Patches • Brugada syndrome • e-Health • Deep learning machine

KEY POINTS

- QT interval prolongation is a marker of risk for life-threatening cardiac arrhythmias. The possibility of its remote monitoring, with the option of prompt intervention, opens major possibilities for prevention.
- There are service providers for remote electrocardiographic monitoring that calculate QTc. The most useful ones are those that transmit data continuously, as they allow physicians to intervene if necessary.
- There are multiple conditions, including patients taking drugs, which might prolong QTc, in which the possibility for early recognition of QTc prolongation would reduce arrhythmic risk.

INTRODUCTION

The times when respected textbooks of electrocardiography could write, "The measurement of the QT interval has no clinical relevance," and remain unchallenged, are over.[1]

Until the 1970s, a prolongation of the QT interval was observed with interest by just a handful of clinicians who had encountered by chance a few dramatic cases of familial sudden death in individuals with bizarre T waves and a marked prolongation of the QT interval.[2] These cases were so odd that even a recognized authority in cardiology as Sam Levine did not dare to report in the *New England Journal of Medicine* his own experience[3] until an almost identical case, involving multiple sudden deaths among siblings, had been published by Anton Jervell in 1957.[2] In the mid-1960s, a short editorial in *The Lancet* brought this issue to a larger public.[4]

The interest for the QT interval exploded in the 1970s when 2 concepts were brought to the attention of clinical cardiologists through publications in journals with a wide readership. The first related to the fact that the number of cases of familiar QT interval prolongation associated with sudden cardiac death in the young (since then called long QT syndrome [LQTS]) were rapidly becoming hundreds and hundreds, thus pointing to a previously unrecognized disease than to a very rare one.[5] The second was the unexpected evidence that among survivors of an acute myocardial infarction, a relatively common cardiovascular disorder, the patients in whom a QT interval prolongation was repeatedly observed on multiple electrocardiograms (ECGs) had a more than double risk of dying

[a] Istituto Auxologico Italiano, IRCCS–Center for Cardiac Arrhythmias of Genetic Origin, Via Pier Lombardo 22, 20135 Milan, Italy; [b] University Hospital Copenhagen, Rigshospitalet, Department of Cardiology, 2142 Blegdamsvej 9, 2100 Copenhagen, Denmark
* Corresponding author.
E-mail address: p.schwartz@auxologico.it

Card Electrophysiol Clin 13 (2021) 523–530
https://doi.org/10.1016/j.ccep.2021.04.010
1877-9182/21/© 2021 Elsevier Inc. All rights reserved.

suddenly.[6] The subsequent replication of these findings by investigators all over the world clinched the acceptance of the concept that a QT prolongation was a major marker of risk for sudden cardiac death.[7]

The next major event was fostered by the unforeseen developments in cardiovascular genetics of the mid-1990s and was brought about by the combination of the initial understanding of the role of cardiac ion channels (and specifically of the repolarizing potassium currents I_{Ks} and I_{Kr}) with the brilliant intuition by Dan Roden that the mechanism underlying the so-called drug-induced LQTS (di-LQTS) was actually a loss of "repolarization reserve" largely owing to a reduction in the I_{Kr} current, which would become manifest with a prolongation of the QT interval.[8] di-LQTS represents still a major problem for the pharmaceutical industry because severe untoward reactions, such as torsades de pointes (TdP), ventricular tachycardia and sudden death observed in just a few patients, have led to the withdrawal from the market of powerful drugs whose development had required large financial investments.[9] These life-threatening events are unacceptable with drugs that are not lifesaving, for example, antibiotics, antidepressants, or anti-inflammatory. The problem is compounded by the fact that, despite a significant genetic component that accounts for approximately 30% of these cases,[10] the occurrence of TdP remains largely unpredictable.[11]

When a patient needs one of the many drugs that reduce or block the I_{Kr} current, the possibility of a close monitoring of the ECG for at least a week becomes important because the individuals who will develop TdP usually react with an excessive QT interval prolongation after just a few days of therapy. Therefore, there is a growing interest in cardiology for devices capable of remote monitoring of QT interval changes and of even short-lasting arrhythmic episodes.

Here, the authors review some of these devices, consider their potential role in the current COVID-19 pandemic, discuss their own experience, present a new multicenter study, and then examine the implications of remote monitoring in various clinical scenarios.

AN OVERVIEW OF CURRENT DEVICES

In recent years, there has been an increased demand for QTc monitoring solutions, and this has been addressed by remote ECG monitoring service providers through the introduction or expansion of services that detect and report QTc prolongation. These services are offered by companies including AliveCor (AliveCor, Inc, San Francisco, CA, USA), BioTelemetry (BioTelemetry, Malvern, PA, USA), and Preventice Solutions (Preventice Solutions Group, Eagan, MN, USA).

In April 2020, AliveCor received Food and Drug Administration clearance for QTc monitoring using their KardiaMobile 6L device in combination with their KardiaPro service. The device and consumer facing subscription service, KardiaCare, are available to consumers without a prescription; however, QTc monitoring is available only to physicians through KardiaPro. The device captures 30-second ECG recordings using 3 electrodes. To capture a recording, the users place their thumbs on 2 front-facing electrodes, while the rear-facing electrode is in contact with their left leg.

The recorded ECG is immediately analyzed producing a classification of normal sinus rhythm, possible atrial fibrillation, bradycardia, tachycardia, or unclassified. Using the smartphone application, a physician can request a QT analysis to be performed on the ECG, and then the recording is sent to an independent diagnostic testing facility where QTc values are determined. Results are generally available within 1 hour.

Both BioTelemetry and Preventice Solutions provide mobile cardiac telemetry (MCT) systems, which may be prescribed by physicians and provide continuous QTc monitoring for up to 30 days. These MCT systems leverage small patch-style monitors (BioTelemetry: MCOT, and Preventice Solutions: BodyGuardian MINI and MINI PLUS) to record the ECG.

BodyGuardian and MCOT are patch monitors recording ECG traces continuously. Traces are sent to a smartphone, and through a specific application, to a server (Cloud) accessible to the clinician using a Web browser. The BioTelemetry MCOT is a 50 × 40 × 9-mm monitor weighting 19 g; it is water-resistant but not waterproof. The latest generation of patch-based technology of the BodyGuardian Remote Monitoring System, called MINI PLUS, is 59 × 30 × 13 mm and weighs 22 g. This system is fully waterproof with an IP67 Intrusion Protection certification allowing complete submersion to 1 m. Both monitors (MCOT and BodyGuardian) can be used for either single-channel patch-based monitoring or 3-channel monitoring when attached to a traditional wired lead set. The BodyGuardian battery on a single charge can operate up to 16 days in Holter mode or up to 7 days in MCT mode. The recorded ECG is transmitted via Bluetooth to a cellular device, which then uploads data to proprietary cloud-based platforms. Such cloud-based platforms run algorithms that measure the QT interval, calculate QTc, and provide support for human overreads and manual QTc measurement as needed. However, whereas the QTc monitoring provided by BodyGuardian has been specifically studied to evaluate its reliability,[12] to the best of the authors' knowledge, no studies are available on the reliability of BioTelemetry MCOT in monitoring QTc.

In recent years, MCT utilization has grown at a rapid pace. High-diagnostic yield[13] and recent hardware and software advancements have helped to drive this increased utilization. Software advancements have improved the performance of automated ECG interpretation with regard to beat detection, beat classification, and rhythm classification[14]; however, a barrier to widespread use of long-term QTc monitoring is the lack of fully automated systems for ECG parameters measurement. Indeed, many other companies offer devices/services that record the ECG [eg, iRhythm (iRhythm Technologies Inc., San Francisco, CA, USA), Apple Watch (Apple Inc, Cupertino, CA, USA)] but do not offer specifically QTc monitoring.

To compensate the lack of fully automated systems for repolarization measurements, constant human overreads, performed at independent diagnostic testing facilities, are required to ensure wave measurement accuracy and consistency.

iRhythm provides an ambulatory cardiac monitoring solution, Zio Service (ZioXT and Zio AT). It consists of a 7-cm patch, water-resistant monitor that acquires and stores the ECG. It has a button that may be pressed by the patient to capture symptomatic events. At the end of the recording period, the monitor patch must be sent to a central monitoring station for a full analysis, and a diagnostic report is generated by certified technicians and sent to the prescribing physician. Also, the Apple Watch system has been recently used in a study to monitor the QTc, even though it does not formally offer this monitoring. Thanks to contacts between the ceramic backplate and the digital crown, by touching with a finger the digital crown for 30 seconds, the user sees a detailed graph of his/her heart rate on the watch. It also indicates the presence of sinus rhythm, atrial fibrillation, and low or high heart rate. The ECG produced in the Apple Health smartphone with the outcome can be e-mailed to a physician. Besides the manual readings, the Apple Watch can also take occasional readings and alert if it detects a rhythm other than sinus rhythm.

State-of-the-art QTc calculation algorithms have been demonstrated to be capable of achieving high accuracy in small patient populations for specific applications.[12] However, no studies have validated automated QTc calculation algorithms using large and diverse patient populations. Perhaps the most commonly used data set for validation of QTc measurement algorithms is

the publicly available Physionet QT Database.[15] This data set consists of 105 ECG records each containing 30 to 50 cardiologist-annotated beats. Because Physionet data sets are publicly available and are referenced within the ANSI/AAMI:EC57 guidelines for testing performance of ECG algorithms, they are widely used for algorithm validation. The QT Database data set contains 105 ECG records, offering some patient diversity; however, it is not representative of any particular pathologic condition, making results difficult to interpret in the context of QTc prolongation. In recent years, cloud-based platforms and widespread use of remote ECG monitoring have enabled researchers in the field of automated ECG interpretation to begin demonstrating algorithm performance using data sets with real-world ECG collected from hundreds of patients.[14,16] Thorough validation is required to drive expanded use and automation in ECG interpretation. These practices must also be applied to drive the development of fully automated wave measurement algorithms and in order to support the increased demand for QTc monitoring solutions.

Among the many studies that, in addition to thorough validation, have used deep learning to create automated ECG interpretation algorithms, two studies[14,16] are the most comprehensive and both used large, diverse, and real-world data sets to train and validate algorithm performance. Applications of deep learning to ECG are still relatively new, but this early work has demonstrated that deep learning has the potential to greatly improve the accuracy of automated ECG interpretation algorithms. In the future, deep learning-based QTc calculation algorithms may enable MCT to be used for fully automated near real-time detection of QTc prolongation. These products would allow for immediate clinical intervention where necessary.

RELEVANT STUDIES TO DATE

Several papers have been published on remote monitoring during the last few years, but just a few have explored the reliability of remote monitoring for the QTc measurements.

The accuracy of AliveCor in QTc calculation was explored in 3 studies.[17–19] Chung and colleagues[17] included only 5 patients on a QTc prolonging drug. Garabelli and colleagues[18] used a modified version (A-SHM) and included 99 healthy volunteers and 20 patients on QTc prolonging drugs. Gropler and colleagues[19] studied 30 pediatric patients. These 3 studies concluded a good accuracy in the determination of QTc prolongation; however, 2 larger studies did not fully reproduce this positive result.[20,21]

In 2015 Chung and colleagues[17] explored the possibility of using the AliveCor heart monitor to oversee the QTc changes in just 5 patients with atrial fibrillation taking dofetilide. They compared an AliveCor tracing for each patient with an ECG performed at approximately the same time that day. No significant difference between the Alive-Cor QTc and ECG QTc was found.

A modified version of the same heart monitor (AliveCor smartphone heart rhythm monitor A-SHM), which allows the recording of 2-lead ECG, was used by Garabelli and colleagues.[18] They compared the AliveCor strips ECG with a 12-lead General Electric ECGs in 99 healthy volunteers and in 20 patients being admitted to the hospital for dofetilide or sotalol loading. Good agreement between the AliveCor monitor and the 12-lead ECG was noted among the healthy subjects. Still good agreement was also noted in the patients, in whom the monitor detected QTc prolongation with a specificity of 97% for QTc greater than 500 milliseconds. Although this may represent on the surface a satisfactory result, it can be argued that with such a high cutoff it would be difficult to find great differences in the measurements, whereas it is more challenging to correctly measure a QT interval that is more modestly prolonged.

A small study of 30 pediatric patients[19] suggested accuracy of the QT interval measurements with AliveCor but a difference greater than 20 milliseconds in QTc was detected in 9 (30%) patients. Although the AliveCor has now been implemented and permits the storage of a 6-lead ECG, this system has the significant limitation of not providing a continuous ECG monitoring, as it is the patient's responsibility to record it and send it to the physician.

Importantly, these results were not entirely reproduced by 2 much larger studies.[20,21] Haberman and colleagues[20] studied 381 subjects, including 123 athletes, 128 healthy students, and 130 ambulatory cardiology clinic patients. By comparing the AliveCor measurements with a standard 12-lead ECG acquired immediately after the smartphone ECG was obtained, the corrected QT interval measurements differed significantly. Koltowski and colleagues[21] compared a standard 12-lead ECG and a Kardia Mobile (AliveCor) system in 100 patients and found that with the AliveCor monitor the QTc values were somewhat shorter.

The authors explored the validity of a remote monitoring system, BodyGuardian.[12] In 20 patients affected by LQTS and all carrying a

disease-causing mutation, they prospectively compared the manual measurements of the QT intervals obtained from the 24-hour 12-lead Holter monitor with the simultaneous evaluation of the QT interval from the ECG patch monitor. The same comparison was also made in 16 controls. Taking into account a total of 351 measurements (219 from LQTS patients and 132 from the healthy controls), the authors found a remarkable correspondence in measurements (QTc was 446 ± 41 and 445 ± 47 milliseconds in the manual measurements and in the BodyGuardian measurements, respectively). Moreover, the number of false positive and false negative measurements was very low (**Fig. 1**). Also, the percentage of disagreement between BodyGuardian measurements and the manual measurements less than 15 milliseconds was acceptable: 57%, 63%, and 54% in the entire population, in controls, and in LQTS patients, respectively. Only 1 out of 36 subjects would have been misclassified: this was a patient with diphasic T waves in lead II, which misled the BodyGuardian measurements. The quality trace recording is guaranteed through a mobile phone alert, and the cardiologist can

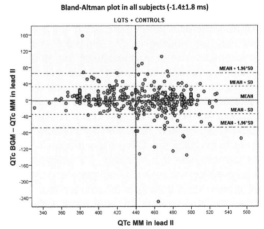

Fig. 1. Dots represent each manually measured QTc in lead II (QTcMM) plotted against each difference between the automated measurements of QTc by Body-Guardian (BGM) and the manually measured QTc (QTc BGM – QTc MM). The vertical red line indicates the upper normal QTc. The closer the plot to 0, the greater is the agreement between the automated and the manual measurements. As indicated by the horizontal red line, the mean value of the plot is close to 0, indicating a high agreement between measurements. SD, standard deviation. (*From* Castelletti S, Dagradi F, Goulene K, et al. A wearable remote monitoring system for the identification of subjects with a prolonged QT interval or at risk for drug-induced long QT syndrome. Int J Cardiol. 2018;266:89-94; with permission)

remotely access the server to view in real-time the clinical data and ECG traces: this ensures the possibility of a prompt recognition of repolarization abnormalities. The subjects involved were comfortable with the device and had no problems with its dimensions, especially compared with the 12-lead Holter monitoring. This article was accompanied by an editorial that commended the investigators "for introducing a highly promising approach using a new patient-friendly wearable ECG monitoring system."[22] It is also worth noting that the accuracy of the BodyGuardian measurements was assessed in moderately prolonged QTc values, in contrast with the AliveCor studies, in which the monitor detected QTc prolongation with a high specificity for QTc greater than 500 milliseconds. The AliveCor system appears to be handy and simple to use; however, its important limitation is that it does not record continuously.

THE ISSUE OF REMOTE MONITORING DURING A PANDEMIC

The problem has become even more important nowadays because of the coronavirus disease 2019 (COVID-19) pandemic, as some of the proposed treatments may prolong QTc, raising safety concerns and logistical problems. Also, the stress and depression related to the COVID-19 pandemic appear to increase the use of antidepressants. In this context, the American College of Cardiology has suggested the use of direct-to-consumer mobile devices for the QTc monitoring of the COVID-19 patients in cases of resources constraints or quarantine.[23] Also the Heart Rhythm Society has suggested the use of mobile cardiac outpatient telemetry when conventional telemetry monitoring is not feasible.[24] Therefore, a device that could monitor the QT interval reliably at distance and inform constantly on its variation is of interest in cardiology.

After a few case reports discussing the potential use of remote monitoring of patients taking QTc prolonging drugs during the COVID-19 pandemic,[25,26] a more extensive study was published. Strik and colleagues[27] compared 12-lead standard ECGs with the smartwatch ECG recording ECG trace (lead I, lead II, and V6) obtained with the use of the Apple Watch Series 4 in 100 patients: compared with the standard ECG, the median absolute error in QTc was somewhat lower in V6 (16 milliseconds) than in lead I and lead II. Bland-Altman analyses revealed a slight overestimation of the QTc with the smartwatch, greater in lead V6 and smallest in lead I. The study demonstrated that the Apple Watch

electrocardiographic tracings allow adequate QT interval measurements, but, similarly to the AliveCor monitor, the Apple Watch Series 4 does not allow a continuous recording of the ECG tracing and real-time remote monitoring.

REMOTE MONITORING FOR LIFE-THREATENING ARRHYTHMIAS

The authors' initial interest in remote monitoring was primarily related to the QT interval[12] and its relation to both the congenital and the acquired forms of LQTS. The general interest for this electrocardiographic interval is largely related to the fact that when its values are abnormal, there is an increased risk for sudden death. On this basis, it is logical to use these devices to explore the possibility of also detecting either life-threatening arrhythmias or markers of electrical instability with the goal of improving risk stratification. The authors' group and the one led by Richard Verrier have pioneered these studies.

A significant hurdle could be represented by the need to select an appropriate study population in which the occurrence of transient, and potentially asymptomatic, arrhythmias might represent a significant risk factor for major cardiac events. Patients with epilepsy and those in whom the diagnosis of idiopathic ventricular fibrillation (IVF) has been made match these criteria.

Verrier's group reviewed the potential for ECG patches to contribute to the monitoring of the risk for sudden cardiac death and concluded that the patches, especially for their ability to track markers of electrical instability, have valuable diagnostic utility and can improve the capacity to guide lifesaving therapy.[28] Verrier's group[29] contributed significantly to the field, also because of the intriguing and novel concept that they proposed: namely, that of the "epileptic heart." The idea is that of a "heart damaged by chronic epilepsy as a result of repeated surges in catecholamines and hypoxemia leading to electrical and mechanical dysfunction." In a small cohort of 12 patients with epilepsy, a condition associated with a definite risk of sudden cardiac death, they looked for T-wave alternans[30,31] either with a Holter recorder alone or simultaneously with 14-day ZioXT extended continuous ECG patch monitor.[29] Among the patients, 6 were newly diagnosed and 6 had chronic epilepsy: significantly higher levels of T-wave alternans were noted in the patients with chronic epilepsy, thus in agreement with the hypothesis that repeated catecholamine discharges would increase cardiac electrical instability. To assess the accuracy of the ZioXT monitor, the baseline and maximum 24-hour

T-wave alternans levels were compared with simultaneous Holter ECG, and the accuracy was equivalent. Despite the limited number of patients, the investigators concluded that the study provides the basis for remote monitoring of ventricular repolarization for sudden cardiac death prevention.[29]

Patients who are resuscitated from a sudden cardiac arrest with documented ventricular fibrillation (VF), and in whom the clinical evaluation does not reveal any known causes of VF, are considered as having IVF.[32] A genetic study in 76 IVF patients has shown that almost 10% of them carry mutations causing catecholaminergic polymorphic ventricular tachycardia (CPVT).[33] It is known that approximately one-third of IVF patients experience new lethal arrhythmias; hence, an ICD is implanted.[32,34] No medical treatment is recommended by the guidelines.[32]

Although the patients are admitted to hospital, they are monitored for any new arrhythmias. However, this monitoring is not focused on repolarization changes and, for instance, there are no systematic approaches to heart rate variability, deceleration capacity, or periodic repolarization dynamics. Nonetheless, these pieces of data might possess important information that could help for risk stratification.

The authors have designed a multicenter international project on IVF patients in which electrocardiographic patterns will be investigated using the new arrhythmia monitor system BodyGuardian MINI Plus. ECG data acquired for several days (up to 14 days) cover a broad variety of different situations like rest, physical activity, sudden posture changes, and sleep. With detailed analysis, one will try to detect not only recurrent arrhythmias and markers of electrical instability but also depolarization/repolarization disorders (eg, QT dispersion, QT prolongation, T-wave alternans, or $T_{peak} - T_{end}$ abnormalities) and changes in autonomic nervous system parameters (heart rate variability, deceleration capacity, periodic repolarization dynamics). Repeating the 14 days of monitoring once a year for 3 years in each patient could provide information on changes over time. The study will aim to determine if (i) electrocardiographic arrhythmia monitor risk markers of future arrhythmia are present, and (ii) there was a concealed diagnosis that caused the cardiac arrest. After the initial arrhythmia monitor data collection, patients will be followed for 3 years.

SUMMARY

This overview on the progress in remote monitoring for repolarization abnormalities and for asymptomatic but threatening ventricular arrhythmias provides a rather straightforward picture.

There are devices capable of following the changes of the QT interval of a patient not only during baseline conditions but likely also during the first weeks of therapy, with drugs having the potential of triggering, at least in genetically predisposed individuals,[10] an arrhythmogenic QTc lengthening. This methodology was found adequate to provide reliable measurements in individuals with both a normal and a congenitally prolonged QT interval, and it seems reasonable to assume that the same reliability will be preserved studying patients with different arrhythmogenic conditions and when the QT interval might prolong in response to drugs blocking the I_{Kr} current.[11] The systems allowing a remote real-time visualization of the ECG traces, with QTc calculation, would have the greatest value in allowing physicians at a distance to intervene, preventing potentially dangerous situations.

There are specific examples of situations where such a remote control would have a significant impact on safety. Among antidepressant and antipsychotic drugs of similar clinical efficacy, there are many that block the I_{Kr} current and which, therefore, are potentially dangerous for patients with a reduced repolarization reserve.[8] Psychiatrists and neurologists often avoid potentially effective drugs because of the well-known risk of TdP ventricular tachycardia. If they would know that the QT interval of their patients could be constantly monitored in the first days or weeks of therapy, they could use the most effective drugs with less concern. Patients affected by Brugada syndrome and showing the risk of increasing type 1 ECG pattern and survivors of IVF[35] are often treated with quinidine as prophylactic treatment.[35,36] However, despite these encouraging supportive pieces of data,[35,36] this practice is limited by the reasonable concern that quinidine, a potent I_{Kr} blocker, could not infrequently dangerously prolong the QT interval and facilitate TdP. The possibility of monitoring repolarization and arrhythmias in IVF survivors and in patients with chronic epilepsy opens new possibilities for arrhythmia prevention. The same concept applies in a situation like the present one with the COVID-19 pandemic: the possibility of monitoring repolarization during home therapy with QT-prolonging drugs could reduce the number of major adverse events.

Last, but not least, this approach could help in the development of new drugs. All too often a potentially very effective drug with some degree of I_{Kr} blocking activity does not enter the market, or it is withdrawn from it, just because of a modest

QTc increase in some healthy volunteers or a few cases of TdP in treated patients, implying major financial losses for drug companies and loss of effective and useful drugs that could benefit many patients.

In all these scenarios, the remote monitoring of QTc and of cardiac arrhythmias for 7 to 14 days could help to identify not only the few subjects at risk and interrupt a therapy that might become dangerous but also the large number of patients who instead could be treated with an effective medication without significant concerns.

CLINICS CARE POINTS

- Whenever the QT interval is markedly prolonged, either in the congenital forms or as a reaction to drugs, there is an increased risk of reentrant arrhythmias, including ventricular fibrillation.
- The increased risk for life-threatening arrhythmias mandates the need for monitoring the QT interval whenever QT-prolonging drugs cannot be avoided and in patients with long QT syndrome and genetically-mediated propensity for arrhythmic events nighttime or at sleep.
- Remote monitoring of the QT interval augments the patients' safety in several situations.

DISCLOSURE

Silvia Castelletti and Bo Gregers Winkel have nothing to disclose; Peter J. Schwartz is a consultant for Preventice Solutions, Inc.

ACKNOWLEDGMENTS

The authors are grateful to Pinuccia De Tomasi for her expert editorial support.

REFERENCES

1. Grant R. Clinical electrocardiography. New York: McGraw Hill; 1957.
2. Jervell A, Lange-Nielsen F. Congenital deaf-mutism, functional heart disease with prolongation of the Q-T interval, and sudden death. Am Heart J 1957;54: 59–68.
3. Levine SA, Woodworth CR. Congenital deaf-mutism, prolonged QT interval, syncopal attacks and sudden death. N Engl J Med 1958;259:412–7.
4. Congenital cardiac arrhythmia. Lancet 1964;284: 26–7.
5. Schwartz PJ, Periti M, Malliani A. The long Q-T syndrome. Am Heart J 1975;89:378–90.
6. Schwartz PJ, Wolf S. QT interval prolongation as predictor of sudden death in patients with myocardial infarction. Circulation 1978;57:1074–7.
7. Wellens HJJ, Schwartz PJ, Lindemans FW, et al. Risk stratification for sudden cardiac death: current status and challenges for the future. Eur Heart J 2014;35:1642–51.
8. Roden DM. Taking the "idio" out of "idiosyncratic": predicting torsades de pointes. Pacing Clin Electrophysiol 1998;21:1029–34.
9. Roden DM. Drug-induced prolongation of the QT interval. N Engl J Med 2004;350:1013–22.
10. Itoh H, Crotti L, Aiba T, et al. The genetics underlying acquired long QT syndrome: impact for genetic screening. Eur Heart J 2016;371456–64.
11. Schwartz PJ, Woosley RL. Predicting the unpredictable: drug-induced QT prolongation and Torsades de Pointes. J Am Coll Cardiol 2016;67:1639–50.
12. Castelletti S, Dagradi F, Goulene K, et al. A wearable remote monitoring system for the identification of subjects with a prolonged QT interval or at risk for drug-induced long QT syndrome. Int J Cardiol 2018;266:89–94.
13. Tsang J-P, Mohan S. Benefits of monitoring patients with mobile cardiac telemetry (MCT) compared with the event or Holter monitors. Med Devices (Auckl) 2013;7:1–5.
14. Teplitzky BA, McRoberts M, Ghanbari H. Deep learning for comprehensive ECG annotation. Heart Rhythm 2020;17(5 Pt B):881–8.
15. Laguna P, Mark RG, Goldberg A, et al. A database for evaluation of algorithms for measurement of QT and other waveform intervals in the ECG. In: Computers in cardiology,1997. IEEE; 1997. p. 673–6.
16. Hannun AY, Rajpurkar P, Haghpanahi M, et al. Cardiologist-level arrhythmia detection and classification in ambulatory electrocardiograms using a deep neural network. Nat Med 2019;25:65–9.
17. Chung EH, Guise KD. QTc intervals can be assessed with the AliveCor heart monitor in patients on dofetilide for atrial fibrillation. J Electrocardiol 2015;48:8–9.
18. Garabelli P, Stavrakis S, Albert M, et al. Comparison of QT interval readings in normal sinus rhythm between a smartphone heart monitor and a 12-lead ECG for healthy volunteers and inpatients receiving sotalol or dofetilide. J Cardiovasc Electrophysiol 2016;27:827–32.
19. Gropler MRF, Dalal AS, Van Hare GF, et al. Can smartphone wireless ECGs be used to accurately assess ECG intervals in pediatrics? A comparison of mobile health monitoring to standard 12-lead ECG. PLoS One 2018;13:e0204403.
20. Haberman ZC, Jahn RT, Bose R, et al. Wireless smartphone ECG enables large-scale screening in

diverse populations. J Cardiovasc Electrophysiol 2015;26:520–6.

21. Koltowski L, Balsam P, Głowczynska R, et al. Kardia Mobile applicability in clinical practice: a comparison of Kardia Mobile and standard 12-lead electrocardiogram records in 100 consecutive patients of a tertiary cardiovascular care center. Cardiol J 2019. https://doi.org/10.5603/CJ.a2019.0001.

22. Verrier RL. The power of the patch: a smart way to track risk for torsades de pointes in congenital and drug-induced long QT syndromes? Int J Cardiol 2018;266:145–6.

23. Lakkireddy DR, Chung MK, Deering TF, et al. Guidance for rebooting electrophysiology through the COVID-19 pandemic from the Heart Rhythm Society and the American Heart Association Electrocardiography and Arrhythmias Committee of the Council on Clinical Cardiology: endorsed by the American College of Cardiology. JACC Clin Electrophysiol 2020;6:1053–66.

24. Varma N, Marrouche NF, Aguinaga L, et al. HRS/EHRA/APHRS/LAHRS/ACC/AHA worldwide practice update for telehealth and arrhythmia monitoring during and after a pandemic. Heart Rhythm 2020;17:e255–68.

25. Chinitz JS, Goyal R, Morales DC, et al. Use of a smartwatch for assessment of the QT interval in outpatients with coronavirus disease 2019. J Innov Card Rhythm Manag 2020;11:4219–22.

26. Gabriels J, Saleh M, Chang D, et al. Inpatient use of mobile continuous telemetry for COVID-19 patients treated with hydroxychloroquine and azithromycin. Heart Rhythm Case Rep 2020;6:241–3.

27. Strik M, Caillol T, Ramirez FD, et al. Validating QT-interval measurement using the Apple Watch ECG to enable remote monitoring during the COVID-19 pandemic. Circulation 2020;142:416–8.

28. Verrier RL, Nearing BD, Pang TD, et al. Monitoring risk for sudden cardiac death: is there a role for EKG patches? Curr Opin Biomed Eng 2019;11:117–23.

29. Pang TD, Nearing BD, Krishnamurthy KB, et al. Cardiac electrical instability in newly diagnosed/chronic epilepsy tracked by Holter and ECG patch. Neurology 2019;93:450–8.

30. Schwartz PJ, Malliani A. Electrical alternation of the T-wave: clinical and experimental evidence of its relationship with the sympathetic nervous system and with the long Q-T syndrome. Am Heart J 1975;89:45–50.

31. Verrier RL, Klingenheben T, Malik M, et al. Microvolt T-wave alternans physiological basis, methods of measurement, and clinical utility–consensus guideline by International Society for Holter and noninvasive electrocardiology. J Am Coll Cardiol 2011;58:1309–24.

32. Priori SG, Wilde AA, Horie M, et al. HRS/EHRA/APHRS Expert consensus statement on the diagnosis and management of patients with inherited primary arrhythmia syndromes. Heart Rhythm 2013;10:1932–63.

33. Leinonen JT, Crotti L, Djupsjöbacka A, et al. The genetics underlying idiopathic ventricular fibrillation: a special role for catecholaminergic polymorphic ventricular tachycardia? Int J Cardiol 2018;250:139–45.

34. Stampe NK, Jespersen CB, Glinge C, et al. Clinical characteristics and risk factors of arrhythmia during follow-up of patients with idiopathic ventricular fibrillation. J Cardiovasc Electrophysiol 2020;31:2677–86.

35. Belhassen B, Glick A, Viskin S. Excellent long-term reproducibility of the electrophysiologic efficacy of quinidine in patients with idiopathic ventricular fibrillation and Brugada syndrome. Pacing Clin Electrophysiol 2009;32:294–301.

36. Belhassen B, Rahkovich M, Michowitz Y, et al. Management of Brugada syndrome: thirty-three-year experience using electrophysiologically guided therapy with class 1A antiarrhythmic drugs. Circ Arrhythm Electrophysiol 2015;8:1393–402.

Atrial Fibrillation Population Screening

Henri Gruwez, MD[a,b,c,d,*], Tine Proesmans, MSc[e], Stijn Evens, MSc[e],
Frederik H. Verbrugge, MD, PhD[f,g,h], Sébastien Deferm, MD[b,c], Jeroen Dauw, MD[b,c],
Rik Willems, MD, PhD[a,d], Pieter Vandervoort, MD, PhD[b,c], Peter Haemers, MD, PhD[a,d],
Laurent Pison, MD, PhD[c]

KEYWORDS

• Atrial fibrillation • Screening • Stroke • Photoplethysmography • Electrocardiogram

KEY POINTS

• Undetected atrial fibrillation (AF) is common and can be detected by screening.
• Clinical AF refers to symptomatic or asymptomatic AF documented by surface ECG, whereas subclinical AF (SCAF) refers to AF detected by screening or continuous monitoring in whom clinical AF is not present.
• Evidence suggests that anticoagulation and rhythm-control therapy for screen-detected AF might lead to better clinical outcomes. The existing evidence is for clinical AF and randomized clinical trials for SCAF are needed.
• The AF detection rate of screening is determined by the population, the tool, the frequency, and the duration of screening. In general, longer and more frequent screening in a population at higher risk for AF results in a higher detection rate.
• Implantable cardiac rhythm devices have the highest AF detection rates. Single-lead ECG and PPG devices are potentially more cost-effective and are more convenient for population-wide screening.

ATRIAL FIBRILLATION DEFINITION, RISK FACTORS, AND EPIDEMIOLOGY

Atrial fibrillation (AF) is the most common sustained cardiac arrhythmia with an estimated prevalence of 2% to 4% and an estimated lifetime risk of 37%.[1,2] The prevalence is expected to rise 2.3 times by 2060 because of the aging of the population, the increasing prevalence of AF risk factors, and intensified efforts to diagnose AF.[3,4] The prevalence of AF increases sharply with age, affecting approximately 5.5% of those greater than or equal to 65 years and exceeding 15% for those greater than or equal to 85 years.[5,6] Other risk factors for AF include male sex, sedentary lifestyle, smoking, obesity, diabetes mellitus, obstructive sleep apnea, arterial hypertension, heart failure, ischemic heart disease, and chronic kidney disease.[7,8] Because most of these risk factors apart from age and gender are to a large extent modifiable, strict management may reduce incident AF.[8]

Symptomatic AF most often presents as palpitations, chest pain, effort intolerance, dizziness, syncope, or sleep disorders, but 50% to 87% of individuals with AF are initially asymptomatic.[8,9] Approximately one-third remains asymptomatic and a large percentage has atypical symptoms, especially in those greater than or equal to

[a] Department of Cardiovascular Sciences, KU Leuven, Leuven, Belgium; [b] Doctoral School of Medicine and Life Sciences, Hasselt University, Hasselt, Belgium; [c] Cardiology Department, Ziekenhuis Oost-Limburg, Schiepse Bos 6, 3600 Genk, Belgium; [d] Cardiology, University hospitals Leuven Herestraat 49, 3000 Leuven, Belgium; [e] Qompium, Kempische steenweg, 303 27, 3500, Hasselt, Belgium; [f] University Hospital Brussels, Avenue du Laerbeek 101, 1090 Jette, Belgium; [g] Faculty of Medicine and Pharmacy, Vrije Universiteit Brussel, Brussels, Belgium; [h] Biomedical Research Institute, Faculty of Medicine and Life Sciences, Hasselt University, Hasselt, Belgium
* Corresponding author. Cardiology, Schiepse Bos 6, Genk 3600, Belgium.
E-mail addresses: Henri.gruwez@zol.be; Henri.gruwez@uzleuven.be

Card Electrophysiol Clin 13 (2021) 531–542
https://doi.org/10.1016/j.ccep.2021.04.009
1877-9182/21/© 2021 Elsevier Inc. All rights reserved.

65 years.[10] As such, between 13% and 35% of people with AF are currently undiagnosed, suggesting the potential yield of intensified screening efforts.[11,12] Detection of AF is hampered by its intermittent and often asymptomatic nature. Based on the duration of its episodes, the AF pattern is currently classified as paroxysmal, persistent, or permanent.[13] However, this classification does not correlate well with the overall time spent in AF (ie, AF burden), which can only be assessed by a continuous monitor device, traditionally an implantable loop recorder (ILR) or pacemaker device.[8]

DIAGNOSIS OF ATRIAL FIBRILLATION

Traditionally, the diagnosis of AF is made on a conventional 12-lead electrocardiogram (ECG) showing no discernible repeating P waves and irregular RR intervals in the absence of high-degree atrioventricular conduction block. Alternatively, the diagnosis can also be made on a greater than or equal to 30-second strip of a single-lead ECG or Holter monitor, following the same criteria.[8,14] The diagnosis of AF on a surface ECG, regardless of the presence of symptoms, is referred to as clinical AF, whereas asymptomatic AF detected by screening or continuous monitoring is referred to as subclinical AF (SCAF) if clinical AF is not present.

WHY TO SCREEN FOR ATRIAL FIBRILLATION?

A plausible advantage of an earlier AF diagnosis through screening is the opportunity to institute oral anticoagulation (OAC) to prevent thromboembolic stroke.[15,16] Clinical AF is associated with a five-fold increased risk of stroke, a three-fold increased risk of heart failure, and a doubling of mortality.[17–19] Moreover, stroke in patients with AF is generally more severe and outcomes are markedly poorer than in patients with sinus rhythm.[20] The stroke risk in patients with clinical AF is reduced by 65% with OAC.[7,21,22]

From all individuals with undiagnosed AF, more than 50% would qualify for current guideline-recommended indications for OAC.[11] Multiple studies have shown increased AF detection rates following a wide variety of screening strategies (**Table 1**).[23–25] In the mHealth Screening To Prevent Strokes (mSToPS) study, screening with a continuous ECG patch for 2 weeks was deployed in a population at risk of AF and stroke with continuous ECG patch monitoring during 2 weeks, yielding 3.9% new AF diagnoses. The 3-year follow-up data of this trial demonstrate a 1% absolute reduction for the combined risk of death, stroke, systemic embolism or myocardial

infarction in the screened group versus matched control subjects (4.5% vs 5.5%).[26,27]

Yet, no data from randomized controlled trials specifically address the risk of stroke and/or death in SCAF; the closest approximation comes from cohort studies of individuals with AF detected incidentally in the absence of symptoms.[28] These studies support the concept that SCAF is associated with an increased risk of stroke or death compared with individuals in sinus rhythm and the presence or absence of symptoms associated with AF is not associated with differences in this risk.[17] However, the absolute risk of patients with SCAF rather than clinical AF is likely lower, making unsure at what AF burden threshold treatments are likely effective.[29,30]

The increased mortality risk associated with AF remains significant after adjustment for stroke risk.[21] Importantly, besides institution of OAC, AF screening may enable early rhythm control and better control of cardiovascular risk factors that contribute to atrial remodeling/cardiomyopathy and development of AF. The latter is a fundamental component in the management AF, as recommended by the 2020 European Society of Cardiology (ESC) guidelines.[8] The benefit of rhythm versus rate control is somewhat controversial and available evidence is conflicting. The Atrial Fibrillation Follow-up Investigation of Rhythm Management (AFFIRM) trial did not show survival benefit between rate and rhythm control.[31] As a result, rhythm control is currently only recommended to reduce AF-related symptoms and improve quality of life in patients with clinical AF.[8] However, the recent EAST trial concluded that early rhythm-control therapy was associated with a lower risk of adverse cardiovascular outcomes among patients with a history of AF shorter than 1 year and cardiovascular conditions.[32] Whether these findings also apply for SCAF remains to be demonstrated. It is known that SCAF strongly predicts clinical AF and early rhythm control might slow down the evolution of atrial myopathy and AF progression.[30,33]

THEORETIC APPROACH TO ATRIAL FIBRILLATION SCREENING STRATEGIES

Fig. 1 displays the diagnostic yield and the effort or cost of screening in relation to the screened population. The true yield of screening is clinical yield or clinical benefit (ie, prevention of adverse outcomes, such as stroke and/or mortality). However, data on the clinical benefit of AF screening are lacking. Instead, screening trials have used new-AF detection rate as a surrogate marker to attain sufficient power. Hence, this rate is used to

Table 1
Selection of atrial fibrillation screening trials, sorted by new atrial fibrillation detection rate

Author; Reference; Year	Study Name; Country	Screening Method; (Confirmation Method)	Screening Period (d)	Setting	Mean Age; Mean CHA$_2$DS$_2$-VASc	Participants Screened	Overall AF Detection Rate	New-AF Detection Rate	
								Control Group	Screening Group
Perez et al,[54] 2019	Apple Heart Study; United States	PPG Smartwatch; (ECG patch)	270	Consumer volunteers	41; NR	419,297	NA	NA	0.036[a]; 0.52[b]
Guo et al,[55] 2019	Huawei Heart Study; China	PPG Smartwatch (12-lead ECG)	180	Consumer volunteers	34.7; NR	187,912	NA	NA	0.12[a]; 0.23[b]
Verbrugge,[72] 2019	DIGITAL-AF 1; Belgium	PPG Smartphone (offline validation)	7	Consumer volunteers	49; NR	12,328	1.1	NA	NR
Proietti et al,[73] 2016	Belgium	Single-lead ECG (12-lead ECG)	SM	Voluntary participants	58.0; NR	65,747	1.4	NA	0.92
Lowres et al,[70] 2014	SEARCH-AF; Australia	Single-lead ECG	SM	Pharmacy	76; 3.3	1000	6.7	NA	1.5
Fitzmaurice et al,[25] 2007	SAFE; UK systematic screening arm	Pulse assessment and 12-lead ECG	SM	Primary health care	73.8; NR	4933	NA	1.04	1.62
Fitzmaurice et al,[25] 2007	SAFE; UK opportunistic screening arm	Pulse palpation and 12-lead ECG	SM	Primary health care	74.0; NR	4933	NA	1.04	1.64
Kemp Gudmundsdottir et al,[37] 2020	STROKESTOP II; Sweden	Single-lead ECG SM, then twice daily[c]	SM, 14[c]	Community invitation (high-risk subgroup is N-terminal pro-B-type	75–76; 3.4	6315	10.5	NR	2.6; 4.4[c]

(continued on next page)

Table 1
(continued)

Author; Reference; Year	Study Name; Country	Screening Method; (Confirmation Method)	Screening Period (d)	Setting	Mean Age; Mean CHA$_2$DS$_2$-VASc	Participants Screened	Overall AF Detection Rate	New-AF Detection Rate	
								Control Group	Screening Group
				natriuretic peptide >125 ng/L)[c]					
Svennberg et al,[24] 2015	STROKESTOP; Sweden	12-lead ECG, then single-lead ECG twice daily	SM, 14	Community invitation	75–76; 3.5	7173	12.3	NA	3.0
Halcox et al,[74] 2017	REHEARSE-AF; United Kingdom	Single-lead ECG, twice weekly	365	Primary health care or research visits	72.6; 3.0	500	NA	1.0	3.7
Steinhubl et al,[26] 2018	mSToPS; United States	Single-lead ECG patch	14	Health plan enrollees	72.4; (3 median)	1366	NA	0.9	3.9
Engdahl et al,[46] 2013	Sweden	12-lead ECG, then single-lead ECG[c] twice daily	SM, 14[c]	Community invitation (high-risk subgroup is CHADS$_2$ ≥2)[c]	75–76; 1.8	848	14.3	NA	5.2
Reiffel et al,[75] 2017	REVEAL AF; United States and Europe	ICM	915	Patients in clinical centers with CHADS$_2$ >2 (or = 2 with other risk factors)	71.5; 2.9	385	NA	NR	40.0

Abbreviations: ICM, insertable cardiac monitor; NA, not applicable; NR, not reported; PPG, photoplethysmography; SM, single measurement.

[a] Confirmed by ECG patch.
[b] Received smartwatch notification.
[c] In a high-risk subgroup.

express the diagnostic yield of screening in **Fig. 1**, which is determined by disease prevalence, test performance, duration, and the frequency of screening.

WHO TO SCREEN FOR ATRIAL FIBRILLATION?

The background risk of the screening population strongly influences the diagnostic yield of screening for AF.[34] These risk factors could theoretically be divided into two categories: characteristics increasing the odds of AF detection, or characteristics increasing the risk of adverse clinical outcome in case of AF detection.[15]

The first category includes risk factors for AF. Because AF increases disproportionally in older adults, age is one of the strongest risk factors for AF.[5] The prevalence of AF in those less than 50 years of age is almost negligible in most populations and may not justify screening in this group.[3] The Apple-Heart study and the Huawei Heart study were conducted in a broad population, with a mean age of 41 years and 35 years. As a result, the AF detection rate was low at 0.036% and 0.12%, respectively (see **Fig. 1**C). By contrast the STROKESTOP study deployed screening targeted to a high-risk population to increase yield and justify more intense screening efforts and expenses. This study was conducted in a population of 75 to 76 years, yielding a total AF detection rate of 12.3% and a new AF detection rate of 3.0%. Risk models, such as CHARGE-AF, can be used to refine the pretest probability of AF based on clinical risk factors (age, race, height, weight, blood pressure, smoking, antihypertensive medication, diabetes, myocardial infarction, and heart failure).[35,36] Other, nonclinical risk factors include: biomarkers, genetic risk factors, and cardiac structural features (eg, left atrial size).[37–40] The STROKESTOP II study used N-terminal pro–B-type natriuretic peptide guided risk stratification to select a high-risk group for intensified screening.[37] Beyond these conventional approaches, experiments with artificial intelligence have predicted AF risk, based on electronic medical health records or ECG data acquired from individuals in sinus rhythm.[41,42]

The second category includes risk factors for stroke if AF is present. The CHA_2DS_2-VASc risk score is used to estimate the risk of stroke in patients with AF and is used by current guidelines to recommend initiation of OAC therapy (using a threshold score of 1 for men and 2 for women).[43,44]

The risk factors (points awarded) in the CHA_2DS_2-VASc risk score consist of congestive heart failure (1 point), hypertension (1 point), age greater than or equal to 75 years (2 points), diabetes

mellitus (1 point), stroke (2 points), vascular disease (1 point), age 65 to 74 years (1 point), and female gender (1 point). Because most risk factors are similar for prediction of AF as for prediction of stroke in AF, there is considerable overlap between these two theoretic approaches. As a result the CHA_2DS_2-VASc risk score also has a high performance for AF prediction and targeted screening to the CHA_2DS_2-VASc risk score can identify individuals who are more likely to display AF on screening and simultaneously to benefit from treatment.[45] The STROKESTOP trial performed single-lead ECG monitoring twice daily during 2 weeks in a Swedish community after excluding patients with a history of AF or AF on initial presentation. Engdahl and colleagues[46,47] reported on an identical screening protocol but excluded individuals with a CHA_2DS_2-VASc risk score lower than 2. As a result, the new-AF detection rate increased from 2.8% to 7.4% and after this trial, the incidence of ischemic stroke declined significantly in the intervention community.

HOW TO SCREEN FOR ATRIAL FIBRILLATION?
Screening Tool

For decades, AF-screening was restricted to opportunistic pulse palpation and 12-lead ECG confirmation. This approach is still recommended by the 2020 ESC guidelines in patients greater than or equal to 65 years.[8] However, new screening tools have been developed and a meta-analysis has demonstrated that blood pressure monitors, pulse oximetry, smartphone applications, and non-12-lead ECG are more accurate to detect AF compared with pulse palpation.[48] The technology used in these devices is categorized as oscillometry, electrocardiography, or photoplethysmography (PPG).

Oscillometry is the technology used by noninvasive blood pressure devices to detect systolic and diastolic blood pressure based on the principle that the arterial wall oscillates when blood flows through an artery during cuff deflation. Blood pressure devices can be adopted to detect AF based on the pulse interval and have been investigated in several screening trials, which reported a sensitivity between 80.6% and 94.4% and specificity between 89.7% and 98.7% for AF detection.[49–51] Automated algorithms can detect AF using oscillometry-based devices without need for manual interpretation, which limits the cost of its application. Large-scale appliance for screening is hampered by the need for additional hardware and need for confirmatory testing.

Electrocardiography measures voltage differences resulting from depolarization and

A Theoretical yield and effort of atrial fibrillation screening

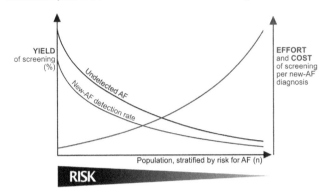

B Diagnostic metrics of a hypothetical atrial fibrillation screening strategy

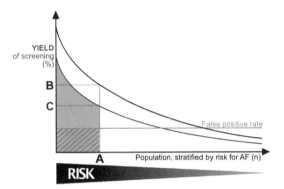

C Positioning of atrial fibrillations screening studies and devices

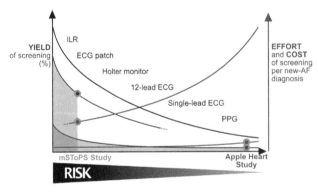

Fig. 1. (*A*) This conceptual graph relates the diagnostic yield of an AF screening program and the effort and cost of screening to the target population. The x-axis represents the screening population stratified by risk for AF (which also correlates to the risk of stroke in case of AF detection). The risk for AF decreases along the x-axis (the individual with the highest risk first, the individual with the second highest risk thereafter, until the entire population is ranked on the x-axis from high-risk to low-risk). The proportion of undetected AF (*black line*) and the diagnostic yield of an AF screening strategy (*blue line*) is represented on the left y-axis. The effort and cost of screening per new-AF diagnosis (*red line*) is represented on the right y-axis. The *black curve* depends only on the characteristics of the population; the *blue curve* and the *red curve* additionally depend on the intrinsic characteristics of the screening strategy (tool, duration, and frequency of screening). (*B*) In a population with size A, the prevalence of unknown AF is B %. A hypothetical screening strategy yields C % new-AF detection rate (true-positive rate). The difference between B and C is the false-negative rate. The false-positive rate is independent of the screened population and therefore remains constant (*orange line*). The area under the curve (AUC) in *green* represents the number of new-AF diagnoses. The AUC in *orange* represents the number of false-positive diagnoses and is directly proportional to the population size. (*C*) The properties of the screening strategy deployed in the mSToPS study and Apple Heart study are displayed as the upper and lower *blue/red lines*, respectively. The mSToPS study targeted a small high-risk population resulting in a high new-AF detection rate and low effort and cost per diagnosis (*brown dots*) and high number of new-AF diagnosis (*brown* AUC). The Apple Heart study targeted a large low-risk population resulting in a low new-AF detection rate and high effort and cost per diagnosis (*blue dots*) and low number of new-AF diagnosis (*blue* AUC) despite screening a large population. A selection of AF screening tools is organized in the graph according to the suggested position in AF screening strategies. From left to right: tools that should be reserved for a high-risk population to tools that can be deployed in the entire population. PPG, photoplethysmography.

repolarization of cardiac muscle tissue. ECG-based devices are classified as invasive (pacemakers, defibrillators, or ILRs) or noninvasive. Invasive devices perform continuous monitoring, and noninvasive tools are classified as continuous or noncontinuous. The noninvasive devices can furthermore be classified according to the number of leads: single-lead (handheld devices, watchbands, and ECG-patches), non-12-lead ECG (Holter monitors and external loop recorders), or conventional 12-lead ECG. Although ECG is considered the most accurate method for AF detection, the diagnostic performance is not uniform across all types of ECG-devices. Twelve-lead ECG remains the gold standard for the diagnosis of an arrhythmia and Holter monitoring for continuous monitoring during 24 to 48 hours. Newer devices, such as ECG patches and ILRs, offer longer continuous monitoring time. These tools are typically analyzed by proprietary automated algorithms and technician supervision with similar diagnostic performance compared with the Holter monitor.[52] Because of the high cost and effort of screening, these devices should be reserved for a population at high risk of AF. The mSToPS trial (see **Fig. 1C, Table 1**) exemplifies such screening strategy.[26] Alternatively, intermittent ECG screening strategies have been performed using a handheld single-lead device in the STROKESTOP trials, or an add-on accessory device to smartphones and smartwatches, used in the Assessment of REmote HEArt Rhythm (REHEARSE-AF) and Screening Education And Recognition in Community pHarmacies of Atrial Fibrillation (SEARCH-AF) trials (see **Table 1**). The diagnostic performance depends on the device, the method of interpretation (single-lead ECG interpretation by physician vs automated algorithm interpretation vs both), the version of the algorithm, and the screened population and should be validated against continuous ECG or ILR. Because of these many factors the reported performance is inconsistent with sensitivity reported from 54.5% to 100% and specificity from 91.9% to 100% for AF detection.[53] The ESC 2020 guidelines and AF-SCREEN international collaboration have summarized the sensitivity as 94% to 98% and 94% to 99% and specificity as 76% to 95% and 92% to 97%, respectively.[8,28] In conclusion, intermittent single-lead devices are high performance screening tools at low-cost, but should be validated in the setting of the screening strategy where they are deployed. The main advantage of single-lead ECG for population-based screening is the ability to provide a verifiable ECG trace and consequently does not require confirmational testing.[28] Yet, the performance of physician interpretation of these traces is unclear. A few studies reported a sensitivity of 91% to 100% and specificity of 87% to 96% for AF detection compared with a 12-lead ECG.[52]

PPG optically obtains changes in capillary blood volume resulting from each systole. PPG technology is exploited by smartphones and smartwatches, assessing the signal on the fingertips or wrist, respectively. The increasing use of smartwatches and ubiquitous spread of smartphones makes PPG an attractive technology for large-scale screening programs. The Apple Heart Study and Huawei Heart study used this technology in smartwatches and demonstrated the scalability because these studies included more than half a million persons collectively.[54,55] The DIGITAL-AF study used a PPG-based smartphone application to screen for AF in more than 12,000 participants who were invited through a local media campaign.[56] The low AF detection rates in these trials are more likely a result from untargeted screening than from poor diagnostic performance. Hence, the currently ongoing HEART LINE study will perform AF-screening with PPG targeted to an elderly population. The accuracy of PPG-based applications varies widely between different algorithms because of the vast number of applications emerging. Considering only four of the most validated algorithms, a systematic review determined an overall sensitivity of 94.2% and specificity of 95.8%.[57] Clear validation studies of PPG algorithms and manual interpretation are needed against simultaneous ECG to establish the use of PPG alone to diagnose AF.

Duration and Frequency of Screening, Defining Screening Intensity

AF can present as an intermittent asymptomatic disorder and therefore remain undetected by a single-timepoint screening strategy. The yield of AF screening increases with duration and frequency of screening.[58] Diederichsen and colleagues[58] simulated different screening strategies in patients with an ILR and risk factors for stroke (**Fig. 2**). In these data, a single 10-second ECG yielded a sensitivity (and negative predictive value) of 1.5% (66%) for AF detection, increasing to 8.3% (67%) for twice-daily 30-second ECGs during 14 days and to 11% (68%), 13% (68%), 15% (69%), 21% (70%), and 34% (74%) for a single 24-hour, 48-hour, 72-hour, 7-day, or 30-day continuous monitoring, respectively.[58] Screening trials that used a single timepoint ECG or pulse palpation have identified AF in 1.4% of the population greater than or equal to 65 years with previously undiagnosed AF.[23] The STROKESTOP study demonstrated the effect of a longer screening duration. Undiagnosed AF was detected in 0.5% with a single 12-lead ECG and increased to 3.0% by additional 2-week single-lead ECG monitoring twice daily.[24] The DIGITAL-AF trial that used PPG to screen for AF similarly found a diagnostic yield of 0.4% with a single heart rhythm assessment that increased to 1.4% during a 7-day screening period.[56]

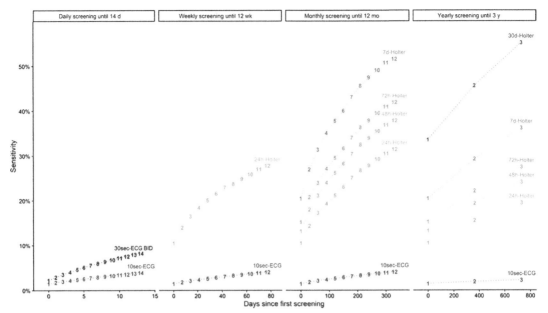

Fig. 2. Sensitivity for detection of atrial fibrillation according to type and number of screenings. The x-axis represents time since first random screening, and the y-axis represents the sensitivity reached after the specified number of consecutive screenings (eg, 1, 2, 3). A 10-second ECG indicates 10-second ECGs taken between 8 AM and 5 PM; 30-second ECG BID, bidaily 30-second ECGs taken at morning and evening; and Holter, any type of continuous monitoring (eg, Holter, R test, event recorder) lasting the specified duration. (*From* Diederichsen SZ, Haugan KJ, Kronborg C, et al. Comprehensive Evaluation of Rhythm Monitoring Strategies in Screening for Atrial Fibrillation: Insights from Patients at Risk Monitored Long Term with an Implantable Loop Recorder. Circulation. 2020;141(19):1510-1522; with permission.)

The extreme of extended screening duration is continuous monitoring. When people with risk factors were continuously monitored with an ILR in the REVEAL AF trial, 40.0% were found to have at least brief AF episodes. This should be distinguished from AF detected by low-frequency intermittent monitoring as performed in the STROKESTOP, DIGITAL-AF, or REVEAL trials because short AF episodes seem to be associated with lower stroke risk.[59,60] Because increasing AF burden correlates with increasing stroke risk, the question remains how much AF mandates OAC therapy. Three ongoing trials, ARTESiA (Apixaban for the Reduction of Thrombo-Embolism in Patients With Device-Detected Sub-Clinical Atrial Fibrillation), Danish LOOP study (Atrial Fibrillation Detected by Continuous ECG Monitoring), and NOAH (Non-vitamin K antagonist Oral anticoagulants in patients with Atrial High rate episodes) aim to answer this question.[61–63] For now, it is known that longer AF duration may result in stroke when comorbidities are less severe, whereas lower AF burdens may result in stroke only when more severe comorbidities are present.[64,65] Hence, screening duration should be in harmony with the disease prevalence and underlying risk for stroke.

PITFALLS OF ATRIAL FIBRILLATION SCREENING

Criticism on widespread implementation of AF screening results from lack of proof of efficiency, possible induction of harm, and insufficient knowledge on AF pathogenesis.[66,67] The number needed to screen (NNS) to prevent stroke or death reflects the screening efficiency. Based on a 0.5% new AF-detection rate and a hypothetical 2% stroke risk reduction with OAC therapy, the NNS is estimated at 10.000, arguing against systematic screening.[66] Yet, AF screening strategies in recent trials have dramatically lowered the NNS by selecting a high-risk population and more accurate screening tools. The mSToPS study yielded a new-AF detection rate of 3.9% in an older population with risk factors using 2-week ECG patch monitoring. In this trial, the NNS decreased to 1282, assuming the hypothetical 2% stroke rate reduction, which is conservative because this population is likely to benefit more from therapy.

Several studies suggest AF screening is cost-effective.[68,69] The SEARCH-AF trial and the STROKESTOP study, both using single-lead ECG devices, estimated an incremental cost-effectiveness ratio of 3142€ and 4614€ per quality-adjusted life-year saved and 15.993€ for preventing one stroke.[70,71] Using technology compatible with consumer devices will further reduce devices costs and likely increase cost-effectiveness.

AF screening can induce harm as a result of anxiety, unwarranted additional testing, or inappropriate therapy in false positives. Screening trials should aim to minimize the identification of individuals who would not benefit from OAC and minimize false-positive results by selecting accurate screening devices and targeting a population high-risk of AF.

Finally, to have an effect on AF pathogenesis and the prevalence of associated adverse events, screening trials should provide a substantial pathway after AF-detection. The ABCCC pathway of the ESC guidelines is such an example.[8]

FUTURE OF ATRIAL FIBRILLATION SCREENING

To determine the most effective screening method, ongoing screening trials aim to determine the impact of screening on stroke reduction. Constructing the most effective method will result from the interplay of the technique, duration, and frequency of screening with the targeted population. There is no population-wide one-fits-all strategy. The highest efficacy is likely to be established in an older population with more risk factors. Ongoing trials target such a population using a variety of screening methods. The VITAL-AF, SAFER, and STROKE-STOP II trials use single-lead ECG devices. The mSToPS and GUARD-AF trials use ECG patch monitoring. The LOOP trial uses ILRs. The HEART LINE study uses PPG and single-lead ECG.

The second question that needs to be answered is what burden of AF is sufficient to justify initiation of OAC. The LOOP, ARTESIA, and NOAH trials will target that issue. At first, these studies will pave the way to various screening strategies, using various tools depending on the target population. In the future, a combination of PPG and single-lead ECG deriving consumer devices will continue to change the landscape of AF screening until every individual is continuously aware of his or her own AF burden. The challenge is to provide answers to these two questions, before the consumer industry surpasses evidence-based clinical knowledge.

CLINICS CARE POINTS

- Atrial fibrillation screening leads to earlier detection of asymptomatic AF.

- Opportunistic screening for AF is recommend in patients of 65 years and older. Systematic screening for AF should be considered in in patients of 75 years and older or patients at high risk of stroke.

- Asymptomatic AF is associated with a higher risk of stroke and mortality and requires treatment based on the thromboembolic risk. Whether this is true for asymptomatic AF detected by screening remains to be demonstrated.

DISCLOSURE

H. Gruwez is supported as predoctoral strategic basic research fellow by the Fund for Scientific Research Flanders. S. Evens and T. Proesmans are employed by Qompium. F.H. Verbrugge has provided strategic advice and academic support to Qompium N.V. F.H. Verbrugge is supported by the Special Research Fund (BOF) of Hasselt University (BOF19PD04). R. Willems reports research funding from Biotronik, Boston Scientific, and Medtronic; and speakers and consultancy fees from Medtronic, Boston Scientific, Biotronik, Abbott, and Microport. P. Vandervoort holds stock in Qompium NV, Belgium. R. Willems is supported as postdoctoral clinical researcher by the Fund for Scientific Research Flanders.

REFERENCES

1. Benjamin EJ, Muntner P, Alonso A, et al. Heart disease and stroke statistics-2019 update: a report from the American Heart Association. Circulation 2019;139(10):e56–528.

2. Staerk L, Wang B, Preis SR, et al. Lifetime risk of atrial fibrillation according to optimal, borderline, or elevated levels of risk factors: cohort study based on longitudinal data from the Framingham Heart Study. BMJ 2018;361:1453.

3. Chugh SS, Havmoeller R, Narayanan K, et al. Worldwide epidemiology of atrial fibrillation: a global burden of disease 2010 study. Circulation 2014; 129(8):837–47.

4. Krijthe BP, Kunst A, Benjamin EJ, et al. Projections on the number of individuals with atrial fibrillation in the European Union, from 2000 to 2060. Eur Heart J 2013;34(35):2746–51.

5. Schnabel RB, Yin X, Gona P, et al. 50 year trends in atrial fibrillation prevalence, incidence, risk factors, and mortality in the Framingham Heart Study: a cohort study. Lancet 2015;386(9989):154–62.

6. Heeringa J, Van Der Kuip DAM, Hofman A, et al. Prevalence, incidence and lifetime risk of atrial fibrillation: the Rotterdam study. Eur Heart J 2006;27(8): 949–53.

7. Staerk L, Sherer JA, Ko D, et al. Atrial fibrillation: epidemiology, pathophysiology, clinical outcomes. Circ Res 2017;120(9):1501–17.

8. Hindricks G, Potpara T, Dagres N, et al. 2020 ESC Guidelines for the diagnosis and management of atrial fibrillation developed in collaboration with the European Association for Cardio-Thoracic Surgery (EACTS): The Task Force for the diagnosis and management of atrial fibrillation of the European Society of Cardiology (ESC) Developed with the special contribution of the European Heart Rhythm Association (EHRA) of the ESC. Eur Heart J 2021;42(5):373–498.

9. Boriani G, Laroche C, Diemberger I, et al. Asymptomatic atrial fibrillation: clinical correlates, management, and outcomes in the EORP-AF Pilot general Registry. Am.J.Med. 2015;128(5):509–18.e2.

10. Healey JS, Connolly SJ, Gold MR, et al. Subclinical atrial fibrillation and the risk of stroke. N Engl J Med 2012;366(2):120–9.

11. Turakhia MP, Shafrin J, Bognar K, et al. Estimated prevalence of undiagnosed atrial fibrillation in the United States. PLoS One 2018;13(4):e0195088.

12. Diederichsen SZ, Haugan KJ, Brandes A, et al. Incidence and predictors of atrial fibrillation episodes as detected by implantable loop recorder in patients at risk: from the LOOP study. Am Heart J 2020;219:117–27.

13. Kirchhof P, Benussi S, Kotecha D, et al. 2016 ESC Guidelines for the management of atrial fibrillation developed in collaboration with EACTS. Eur J Cardiothorac Surg 2016;50(5):e1–88.

14. January CT, Wann LS, Alpert JS, et al. 2014 AHA/ACC/HRS guideline for the management of patients with atrial fibrillation: executive summary: a report of the American College of Cardiology/American Heart Association task force on practice guidelines and the Heart Rhythm Society. Circulation 2014;130(23):2071–104.

15. Mairesse GH, Moran P, Van Gelder IC, et al. Screening for atrial fibrillation: a European Heart Rhythm Association (EHRA) consensus document endorsed by the Heart Rhythm Society (HRS), Asia Pacific Heart Rhythm Society (APHRS), and Sociedad Latinoamericana de Estimulación Cardíaca y Electrofisiolog. Europace 2017;19(10):1589–623.

16. Dobreanu D, Svendsen JH, Lewalter T, et al. Current practice for diagnosis and management of silent atrial fibrillation: results of the European Heart Rhythm Association survey. Europace 2013;15(8):1223–5.

17. Wolf PA, Abbott RD, Kannel WB. Atrial fibrillation as an independent risk factor for stroke: the Framingham study. Stroke 1991;22(8):983–8.

18. Mcallen PM, Marshall J. Cardiac dysrhythmia and transient cerebral ischaemic attacks. Lancet 1973;301(7814):1212–4.

19. Chugh SS, Blackshear JL, Shen WK, et al. Epidemiology and natural history of atrial fibrillation: clinical implications. J Am Coll Cardiol 2001;37(2):371–8.

20. Jørgensen HS, Nakayama H, Reith J, et al. Acute stroke with atrial fibrillation. Stroke 1996;27(10):1765–9.

21. Hart RG, Pearce LA, Aguilar MI. Meta-analysis: antithrombotic therapy to prevent stroke in patients who have nonvalvular atrial fibrillation. Ann Intern Med 2007;146(12):857–67. Available at: www.annals.org. Accessed December 3, 2020.

22. Freedman B, Potpara TS, Lip GYH. Stroke prevention in atrial fibrillation. Lancet 2016;388(10046):806–17.

23. Lowres N, Neubeck L, Redfern J, et al. Screening to identify unknown atrial fibrillation: a systematic review. Thromb Haemost 2013;110(2):213–22.

24. Svennberg E, Engdahl J, Al-Khalili F, et al. Mass screening for untreated atrial fibrillation the STROKESTOP study. Circulation 2015;131(25):2176–84.

25. Fitzmaurice DA, Hobbs FDR, Jowett S, et al. Screening versus routine practice in detection of atrial fibrillation in patients aged 65 or over: cluster randomised controlled trial. Br Med J 2007;335(7616):383–6.

26. Steinhubl SR, Waalen J, Edwards AM, et al. Effect of a home-based wearable continuous ECG monitoring patch on detection of undiagnosed atrial fibrillation the mSToPS randomized clinical trial. JAMA 2018;320(2):146–55.

27. Steinhubl SR, Waalen J, Anirudh Sanyal AM, et al. 3-year Clinical Outcomes in a Nationwide Pragmatic Clinical Trial Of Atrial Fibrillation Screening - mHealth Screening To Prevent Strokes (mSToPS). In: As Presented at 2020 AHA Annual Meeting, Scientific Session. American Heart Association Inc.; Dallas, TX, USA November 13–17, 2020.

28. Freedman B. Screening for atrial fibrillation. Circulation 2017;135(19):1851–67.

29. Jones NR, Taylor CJ, Hobbs FDR, et al. Screening for atrial fibrillation: a call for evidence. Eur Heart J 2020;41(10):1075–85.

30. Mahajan R, Perera T, Elliott AD, et al. Subclinical device-detected atrial fibrillation and stroke risk: a systematic review and meta-analysis. Eur Heart J 2018;39(16):1407–15.

31. Kamp O, Kingma T, Sc M, et al. A comparison of rate control and rhythm control in patients. N Engl J Med 2002;347(23):1825–33. Available at: www.nejm.org.

32. Kirchhof P, Camm AJ, Goette A, et al. Early rhythm-control therapy in patients with atrial fibrillation. N Engl J Med 2020;383(14):1305–16.

33. Reddy YNV, Obokata M, Verbrugge FH, et al. Atrial dysfunction in patients with heart failure with preserved ejection fraction and atrial fibrillation. J Am Coll Cardiol 2020;76(9):1051–64.

34. Rose G, Barker JP. London, medical commission on accident prevention. J Accid Anal Prev 1976;8(43):1417–8.

35. Alonso A, Roetker NS, Soliman EZ, et al. Prediction of atrial fibrillation in a racially diverse cohort: the multi-ethnic study of atherosclerosis (mesa). J Am Heart Assoc 2016;5(2):e003077.

36. Alonso A, Krijthe BP, Aspelund T, et al. Simple risk model predicts incidence of atrial fibrillation in a racially and geographically diverse population: the CHARGE-AF consortium. J Am Heart Assoc 2013;2(2):e000102.

37. Kemp Gudmundsdottir K, Fredriksson T, Svennberg E, et al. Stepwise mass screening for atrial fibrillation using N-terminal B-type natriuretic peptide: the STROKESTOP II study. Europace 2020;22(1):24–32.

38. Weng LC, Preis SR, Hulme OL, et al. Genetic predisposition, clinical risk factor burden, and lifetime risk of atrial fibrillation. Circulation 2018;137(10):1027–38.

39. Gardner JD, Skelton WP, Khouzam RN. Is it time to incorporate the left atrial size to the current stroke risk scoring systems for atrial fibrillation? Curr Probl Cardiol 2016;41(9–10):251–9.

40. Bruun Pedersen K, Madsen C, Sandgaard NCF, et al. Left atrial volume index and left ventricular global longitudinal strain predict new-onset atrial fibrillation in patients with transient ischemic attack. Int J Cardiovasc Imaging 2019;35:1277–86.

41. Hulme OL, Khurshid S, Weng LC, et al. Development and validation of a prediction model for atrial fibrillation using electronic health records. JACC Clin Electrophysiol 2019;5(11):1331–41.

42. Attia ZI, Noseworthy PA, Lopez-Jimenez F, et al. An artificial intelligence-enabled ECG algorithm for the identification of patients with atrial fibrillation during sinus rhythm: a retrospective analysis of outcome prediction. Lancet 2019;394(10201):861–7.

43. Olesen JB, Lip GYH, Hansen ML, et al. Validation of risk stratification schemes for predicting stroke and thromboembolism in patients with atrial fibrillation: nationwide cohort study. Bmj 2011;342(7792):320.

44. Lip GYH, Nieuwlaat R, Pisters R, et al. Refining clinical risk stratification for predicting stroke and thromboembolism in atrial fibrillation using a novel risk factor-based approach: the Euro Heart Survey on atrial fibrillation. Chest 2010;137(2):263–72.

45. Saliba W, Gronich N, Barnett-Griness O, et al. Usefulness of CHADS2 and CHA2DS2-VASc scores in the prediction of new-onset atrial fibrillation: a population-based study. Am J Med 2016;129(8):843–9.

46. Engdahl J, Andersson L, Mirskaya M, et al. Stepwise screening of atrial fibrillation in a 75-year-old population: implications for stroke prevention. Circulation 2013;127(8):930–7.

47. Engdahl J, Holmén A, Rosenqvist M, et al. A prospective 5-year follow-up after population-based systematic screening for atrial fibrillation. Europace 2018;20(FI3):f306–11.

48. Taggar JS, Coleman T, Lewis S, et al. Accuracy of methods for detecting an irregular pulse and suspected atrial fibrillation: a systematic review and meta-analysis. Eur J Prev Cardiol 2016;23(12):1330–8.

49. Quinn FR, Gladstone DJ, Ivers NM, et al. Diagnostic accuracy and yield of screening tests for atrial fibrillation in the family practice setting: a multicentre cohort study. C Open 2018;6(3):E308–15.

50. Kearley K, Selwood M, Van Den Bruel A, et al. Triage tests for identifying atrial fibrillation in primary care: a diagnostic accuracy study comparing single-lead ECG and modified BP monitors. BMJ Open 2014;4(5):e004565.

51. Chan PH, Wong CK, Pun L, et al. Diagnostic performance of an automatic blood pressure measurement device, Microlife WatchBP Home A, for atrial fibrillation screening in a real-world primary care setting. BMJ Open 2017;7(6):1–6.

52. Zungsontiporn N, Link MS. Newer technologies for detection of atrial fibrillation. BMJ 2018;363:k3946.

53. Wong KC, Klimis H, Lowres N, et al. Diagnostic accuracy of handheld electrocardiogram devices in detecting atrial fibrillation in adults in community versus hospital settings: a systematic review and meta-analysis. Heart 2020;106(16):1211–7.

54. Perez MV, Mahaffey KW, Hedlin H, et al. Large-scale assessment of a smartwatch to identify atrial fibrillation. N Engl J Med 2019;381(20):1909–17.

55. Guo Y, Wang H, Zhang H, et al. Mobile photoplethysmographic technology to detect atrial fibrillation. J Am Coll Cardiol 2019;74(19):2365–75.

56. Verbrugge FH, Proesmans T, Vijgen J, et al. Atrial fibrillation screening with photo-plethysmography through a smartphone camera. Europace 2019;21(8):1167–75.

57. O'Sullivan JW, Grigg S, Crawford W, et al. Accuracy of smartphone camera applications for detecting atrial fibrillation: a systematic review and meta-analysis. JAMA Netw Open 2020;3(4):e202064.

58. Diederichsen SZ, Haugan KJ, Kronborg C, et al. Comprehensive evaluation of rhythm monitoring strategies in screening for atrial fibrillation: insights from patients at risk monitored long term with an implantable loop recorder. Circulation 2020;141(19):1510–22.

59. Van Gelder IC, Healey JS, Crijns HJGM, et al. Duration of device-detected subclinical atrial fibrillation and occurrence of stroke in ASSERT. Eur Heart J 2017;38(17):1339–44.

60. Go AS, Reynolds K, Yang J, et al. Association of burden of atrial fibrillation with risk of ischemic stroke

in adults with paroxysmal atrial fibrillation: the KP-RHYTHM study. JAMA Cardiol 2018;3(7):601–8.

61. Lopes RD, Alings M, Connolly SJ, et al. Rationale and design of the apixaban for the reduction of thrombo-embolism in patients with device-detected sub-clinical atrial fibrillation (ARTESiA) trial. Am Heart J 2017;189:137–45.

62. Diederichsen SZ, Haugan KJ, Køber L, et al. Atrial fibrillation detected by continuous electrocardiographic monitoring using implantable loop recorder to prevent stroke in individuals at risk (the LOOP study): Rationale and design of a large randomized controlled trial. Am Heart J 2017;187:122–32.

63. Kirchhof P, Blank BF, Calvert M, et al. Probing oral anticoagulation in patients with atrial high rate episodes: rationale and design of the Non–vitamin K antagonist Oral anticoagulants in patients with Atrial High rate episodes (NOAH–AFNET 6) trial. Am Heart J 2017;190:12–8.

64. Kochav SM, Reiffel JA. Detection of previously unrecognized (subclinical) atrial fibrillation. Am J Cardiol 2020;127:169–75.

65. Kaplan RM, Koehler J, Ziegler PD, et al. Stroke risk as a function of atrial fibrillation duration and CHA2DS2-VASc score. Circulation 2019;140(20):1639–46.

66. Mandrola J, Foy A, Naccarelli G. Screening for atrial fibrillation comes with many snags. JAMA Intern Med 2018;178(10):1296–8.

67. Berge T. Wilson and Jungner would not approve of screening for atrial fibrillation. BMJ 2019;365:l1416.

68. Jacobs MS, Kaasenbrood F, Postma MJ, et al. Cost-effectiveness of screening for atrial fibrillation in primary care with a handheld, single-lead electrocardiogram device in The Netherlands. Europace 2018;20(1):12–8.

69. Welton NJ, McAleenan A, Thom HHZ, et al. Screening strategies for atrial fibrillation: a systematic review and cost-effectiveness analysis. Health Technol Assess (Rockv) 2017;21(29): vii–235.

70. Lowres N, Neubeck L, Salkeld G, et al. Feasibility and cost-effectiveness of stroke prevention through community screening for atrial fibrillation using iPhone ECG in pharmacies: the SEARCH-AF study. Thromb Haemost 2014;111(6):1167–76.

71. Aronsson M, Svennberg E, Rosenqvist M, et al. Cost-effectiveness of mass screening for untreated atrial fibrillation using intermittent ECG recording. Europace 2015;17(7):1023–9.

72. Verbrugge FH, Proesmans T, Vijgen J, et al. Atrial fibrillation screening with photo-plethysmography through a smartphone camera. Europace 2019; 21(8):1167–75.

73. Proietti M, Mairesse GH, Goethals P, et al. A population screening programme for atrial fibrillation: a report from the Belgian Heart Rhythm Week screening programme. Europace 2016;18(12): 1779–86.

74. Halcox JPJ, Wareham K, Cardew A, et al. Assessment of remote heart rhythm sampling using the AliveCor heart monitor to screen for atrial fibrillation the REHEARSE-AF study. Circulation 2017;136(19): 1784–94.

75. Reiffel JA, Verma A, Kowey PR, et al. Incidence of previously undiagnosed atrial fibrillation using insertable cardiac monitors in a high-risk population: the REVEAL AF study. JAMA Cardiol 2017;2(10): 1120–7.

The Role of Artificial Intelligence in Arrhythmia Monitoring

Konstantinos C. Siontis, MD, Paul A. Friedman, MD*

KEYWORDS

- Artificial intelligence • Machine learning • Electrocardiography • Arrhythmia • Monitoring

KEY POINTS

- Vast amounts of digital data are generated from various prescribed and consumer-facing rhythm recording and monitoring devices.
- Artificial intelligence (AI) methods with progressively increasing sophistication have been applied to rhythm monitoring data over the past decade.
- AI-enabled analysis of rhythm monitoring data can facilitate the large-scale deployment of highly precise, consumer-facing, real-time applications for health and disease monitoring with actionable information.
- Global emphasis on digital transformation across all resource settings, advances in storage and secure exchange of data across institutions, coordinated engagement of regulatory and industry partners, cost reductions, and clear demonstration of outcome improvements that are important to patients and other stakeholders will help drive meaningful and large-scale innovation.

INTRODUCTION

The management of cardiac rhythm disorders has been revolutionized by the progress in hardware and software for the recording, storage, processing, and transfer of electrophysiologic signals. From the standard 12-lead electrocardiogram (ECG) that has been a sine qua non in the cardiologist's toolbox for many decades, to the real-time, consumer-facing miniaturized wearable ECG devices, we have witnessed a broadening of the capabilities and scope of rhythm monitoring tools that are impacting the daily lives of millions of people worldwide, both in health and disease. Computer-based algorithmic analysis of the ECG has been used for a long time based on predefined rules and manual feature recognition. However, in more recent years, the availability of vast amounts of digitally acquired and stored electrophysiologic signal data coupled with adaptation of powerful artificial intelligence (AI) analytics on these signals are creating a path toward efficient, accurate, and scalable cardiac disease phenotyping, rhythm determination, and arrhythmia monitoring. In this review, we present an overview of the current state and future of the role of AI in arrhythmia monitoring.

PRIMER ON MACHINE LEARNING AND DEEP LEARNING

In broad terms, AI is the field of computer science dedicated to the theory and development of automated computer systems and software that can complete tasks in a humanlike manner. Machine learning (ML) refers to the large subfield of AI in which models and algorithms are trained to perform a particular task with increasingly good performance when the model is exposed to a repeated learning process. The vast amount of data generated through the expanding array of rhythm monitoring technologies offers a rich substrate for ML applications. Training of ML models can be performed with various approaches, from

Department of Cardiovascular Medicine, Mayo Clinic, 200 First Street Southwest, Rochester, MN 55905, USA
* Corresponding author.
E-mail address: friedman.paul@mayo.edu

Card Electrophysiol Clin 13 (2021) 543–554
https://doi.org/10.1016/j.ccep.2021.04.011
1877-9182/21/© 2021 Elsevier Inc. All rights reserved.

the traditional logistic regression, which is ubiquitous in predictive modeling in the medical literature, to random forest models, reinforcement learning. and the more advanced supervised and unsupervised approaches. The data discussed in this review focuses largely on supervised and unsupervised learning methods.

In supervised learning, data require a label when the model is trained. For example, developing an ML model for predicting atrial fibrillation (AF) based on ECGs recorded during sinus rhythm required that each digital sinus rhythm ECG was labeled as belonging to a patient with or without a known history of documented AF.[1] During training, the computer is repeatedly exposed to labeled specimens, and over time adapts the mathematical weights in its many "neurons" to minimize an error function, and thus correctly classify an unknown specimen presented to it after training is complete. In most examples, specimens are labeled by humans ("this ECG is from a patient with atrial fibrillation," "this picture contains a dog"), in order to train the network: a labor-intensive process when tens of thousands or millions of records are required for training. This puts enormous value on labeled data, and hence the concept that "data is the new oil." It also may impede data sharing due to data value, patient privacy, and intellectual property concerns, potentially limiting independent validation and introducing challenges for peer review. New strategies to automatically create labels for training are under development but may not ameliorate all of these challenges.

In unsupervised learning approaches, which have been less utilized in medicine, data labeling is not required, but rather a model is trained to detect relationships within the data itself without direct human input. Cluster analytical approaches are common examples of unsupervised learning. Unsupervised learning models have the advantage of a lower risk of random or systematic error introduced by a human at the time of labeling. An example of unsupervised cluster analysis is demonstrated in the study by Levy and colleagues[2] in which investigators sought to assess patterns of drug dosing adjustments and to develop ML approaches to identify successful drug initiation in patients undergoing inpatient dofetilide treatment. In that study, the performance of the unsupervised model exceeded that of a supervised approach. In the same study, reinforcement learning approaches were also implemented in which the model is trained based on a reward system so that a correct decision at each step (such as choosing the dose of dofetilide) is awarded with the desired endpoint (such as successful dofetilide initiation). The continuous process of updating inputs and endpoints leads to the optimal reinforcement learning model.[3]

Deep learning is a subfield of ML that uses multilayer networks to identify an association between input and output data. In these deep models, the representation of the input data is learned by the network without human feature selection, therefore the model representation is agnostic. For example, to train a network to identify left ventricular dysfunction from an ECG, each ECG is labeled as to whether or not it is associated with a low ejection fraction (a human effort), but the ECG features (eg, QRS duration, T-wave characteristics) are selected by the network and not knowable to humans. As a result, networks are considered black boxes: their inner workings remain opaque to human understanding. Convolutional neural networks (CNNs) are among the most common type of networks and they are composed of feature extraction layers (using convolutional filters) followed by mathematical modeling layers to classify an image. In the example of AI analysis on the ECG, convolutions can be performed on the temporal (or horizontal) axis representing the timeseries from each lead, the vertical axis representing the voltage in a specific time point, or both. Hence, CNNs learn a representation of input data in an agnostic way and without the risk of bias introduced by human feature selection. Importantly, although model creation typically requires vast data sets and computing power, once created, the models can run with limited resources, effectively on a smartphone. For more in-depth descriptions of AI and ML methods particularly pertaining to cardiovascular medicine applications we refer the reader to several recent comprehensive reviews.[4–6]

SIGNAL SOURCES AND ACQUISITION

Standard and ambulatory ECG data are acquired and stored in large amounts in daily clinical practice. These ECG datasets coupled with exponential growth in computational power have enabled the development of ML models using the statistical power of large sample sizes (**Table 1**). Technical advancements have reduced the size and increased battery longevity of ambulatory heart rate and rhythm monitors, and have made it possible to integrate them in wristband fitness trackers (such as FitBit), chest wall patches (eg, BodyGuardian, Zio monitor), smartwatches (Apple Watch), smartphone-based applications (such as AliveCor KardiaMobile), belts, rings, or even "smart" wearable garments, including shoes and underwear.[7,8] These tools have gained popularity both among clinicians and patients, as they provide a wealth of useful information to clinicians

Table 1
Major contemporary ECG databases used in the development of deep-learning AI-ECG applications

Dataset	Country	Years of Enrollment	Number of Patients Included	ECG Type	Conditions, Outcomes and Scope of Application	References
Minas Gerais/Brazil from the Telehealth Network of Minas Gerais	Brazil	2010–2018	1,676,384	12-lead	Automated ECG interpretation	43
Mayo Clinic	USA	1994–2017	449,380	12-lead	Automated ECG interpretation; LV dysfunction; silent AF; hypertrophic cardiomyopathy; age, sex, race/ethnicity; serum potassium	1,10–12,34,44–47
Geisinger	USA	1984–2019	253,397	12-lead	Overall survival	48
Huazhong University, Wuhan	China	2012–2019	71,520	12-lead	Automated ECG interpretation	33
iRhythm Technologies Inc/Stanford	USA	2013–2017	53,549	Single-lead, ambulatory ECG monitoring	Classification of 12 rhythm types	29
University of California, San Francisco	USA	2010–2017	36,186 (ECGs)	12-lead	LV mass; LA volume; mitral e-prime; pulmonary hypertension; HCM; amyloidosis; mitral prolapse	20
Health eHeart Study	Multinational	2016–2017	9750	Single-lead, smartwatch-based	Passive AF detection	24
CPSC2018	China	2018	6877	12-lead	Classification of 9 rhythm types	49
Cleveland Clinic	USA	2003–2012 & 2017–2018	946	12-lead	Cardiac resynchronization therapy response	50

Abbreviations: AF, atrial fibrillation; AI, artificial intelligence; ECG, electrocardiogram; HCM, hypertrophic cardiomyopathy; LV, left ventricle.
From Siontis KC, Noseworthy PA, Attia ZI and Friedman PA. Artificial intelligence-enhanced electrocardiography in cardiovascular disease management. Nat Rev Cardiol. 2021; with permission.

but also to patients who are able to self-monitor their rhythm abnormality. The rapid rise in the use of wearable, consumer-facing rhythm technologies in the past decade has expanded the data sources of digital ECG signals for AI analysis. Other potential signal sources that may be used in various ML applications include inpatient telemetry recordings and cardiac implanted electronic device data.

Traditionally, wearable heart rate monitoring technologies have been based on passive pulse photoplethysmography (PPG) in which light at a frequency absorbed by hemoglobin is projected onto skin to detect changes in blood flow to determine the pulse rate. In addition, assessment of pulse irregularity permits arrhythmia detection, but in the absence of an electrocardiographic record the ability to differentiate arrythmia from artifact is limited.[9] More recently, interest has shifted from surrogate rhythm assessment via pulse PPG to recording of single-lead or multi-lead bipolar ECG signals acquired from wearable device electrodes in contact with the skin. A common strategy is to use the PPG to passively detect a potential arrhythmia, and then at that time to indicate to the device wearer to record an ECG, which typically requires active user participation. ECG signals are attractive for AI analysis. Wearables provide prolonged continuous or intermittent data for analysis, whereas the 12-lead ECG is acquired in standardized manner that may facilitate analysis. However, ECG data from wearables is usually acquired in less controlled settings than the standard 12-lead ECG, making them susceptible to noise that may hamper the accuracy of developed algorithms. Despite existing methods for filtering of high-frequency and low-frequency artifact from ambulatory recordings, it may be impossible to generate completely noise-free data from wearable devices. The signal-to-noise ratio varies across rhythm-recording devices, patients, recording location, body position and activity during recording, and ambient electromagnetic noise, among other confounders. This heterogeneity in signal recording is difficult to predict and standardize, and thus correct for, but prolonged recording times and noise detection may permit utilization of signals only during intervals with a higher signal-to-noise ratio, and the sheer volume of data acquired may permit compensation for its inferior quality.

APPLYING ARTIFICIAL INTELLIGENCE TO THE ELECTROCARDIOGRAM: THE ARTIFICIALLY INTELLIGENT ELECTROCARDIOGRAM

The availability of large sets of digitally stored ECGs combined with well-phenotyped cohorts of individuals with detailed EMR data has led to a dramatic growth in the use of CNNs for the detection of cardiac disease from the ECG alone (see **Table 1**). Our group at Mayo Clinic has developed CNNs in which the input is a standard digital ECG and the outputs are probability scores for the presence of conditions such as left ventricular systolic dysfunction (LVSD),[10] silent AF,[1] hypertrophic cardiomyopathy (HCM),[11] amyloid heart disease, pulmonary hypertension, or valvular heart disease. We have also developed models for the determination of sex and age.[12] The AI-ECG age may be a surrogate for physiologic age, hence it may be associated with overall survival more closely compared with chronologic age. The discrepancy between chronologic and AI-ECG (physiologic) age (ie, the age gap) may be a marker of physical fitness, or lack thereof, and therefore predictive of long-term mortality. Early data suggest it correlates with vascular age.[13]

Applying multiple AI algorithms simultaneously on a single ECG can be viewed as ECG-based deep cardiac phenotyping to characterize the risk of silent or undiagnosed cardiac disease, or determine overall prognosis and target preventive or therapeutic interventions with precision. Many of these CNNs have demonstrated good performance when applied on single-lead ECG recordings, which makes it possible for them to be integrated into point of care, and in some instances, smartphone or wearable ECG technologies for real-time implementation. However, their utility and downstream effects require validation. A few specific examples of the developed CNN models are discussed in the following.

Detection of Left Ventricular Systolic Dysfunction

Using data from ECGs acquired within days of an echocardiogram in approximately 45,000 patients, an ECG-based CNN was developed to identify LVSD (defined as LVEF ≤35%).[10] When tested in an independent cohort of more than 50,000 patients, the CNN detected LVSD with precision, with an area under the receiver-operating characteristic curve (AUC) of 0.93 with corresponding sensitivity, specificity, and accuracy of 93%, 86.3%, and 85.7%, respectively. Importantly, patients with seemingly false positive detections of LVSD based on the AI-ECG CNN were 4 times more likely to develop future LVSD compared with those with a negative screen. This suggests that the CNN may be able to detect early stages of LVSD even before the LVEF declines by echocardiography. Mechanistically, this may reflect early myopathic processes that interfere with channel function or gap junctions and cell-to-cell conduction, resulting in multiple, nonlinear, subclinical ECG changes that are underappreciated by human readers but detected by a trained neural network. This and other algorithms have been integrated in the electronic health record for point-of-care application in our institution (**Fig. 1**).The algorithm has also demonstrated high accuracy in detecting low LVEF when applied to a single ECG lead thus permitting its implementation with smartphone-based or stethoscope-based electrodes. The US Food and Drug Administration (FDA) recently issued an emergency use authorization for the detection of LVSD as a potential complication of the COVID-19 infection using this AI-ECG algorithm integrated in a digital stethoscope (Eko Devices, Inc, San Francisco, CA).[14]

anticoagulation is indicated; in its absence, anti-platelet agents are used.[16,17] We have recently developed a CNN to predict AF based on a standard 12-lead ECG obtained during sinus rhythm using a cohort of more than 120,000 patients.[1] The model was validated in separate testing cohorts. Patients with at least 1 ECG showing AF within 30 days after the sinus rhythm ECG were classified as positive for AF. In the testing dataset, the AUC for AF detection was 0.87, with a sensitivity of 79.0%, and a specificity of 79.5%. In a recent evaluation, we have demonstrated that the AF AI-ECG algorithm was an independent predictor of incident clinical AF diagnosis in a community-based cohort.[18] This AI tool essentially converts a routine 10-second ECG from a spot tracing into a prolonged rhythm monitoring tool (**Fig. 2**). This algorithm may facilitate targeted AF

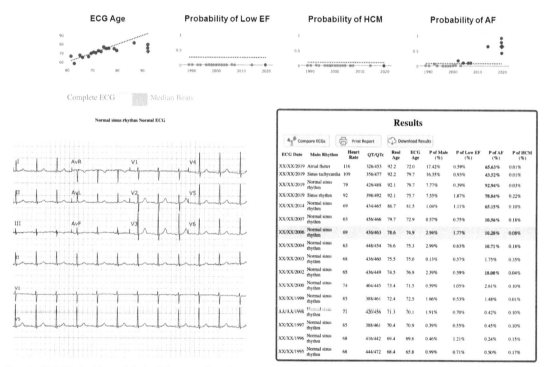

Fig. 1. AI-ECG dashboard linked from within the electronic health record for point-of-care application. This patient with cryptogenic stroke had an elevated probability of silent AF that predated the clinical onset of atrial flutter. (*Adapted from* Siontis KC, Noseworthy PA, Attia ZI and Friedman PA. Artificial intelligence-enhanced electrocardiography in cardiovascular disease management. Nat Rev Cardiol. 2021; with permission).

Detection of Silent Atrial Fibrillation

The value of screening for AF in asymptomatic individuals remains a matter of debate and there is currently insufficient data to recommend routine AF screening in general populations.[15] However, the detection of AF in patients with cryptogenic stroke guides therapy: when AF is present,

screening and surveillance, and may also have a particularly useful role in the evaluation of patients with embolic stroke of undetermined source (ESUS). A spot ECG powered with AI analysis may obviate the need for cumbersome and costly long-term ambulatory rhythm monitors, or help target these interventions to the most high-risk individuals. We have previously reported the case of

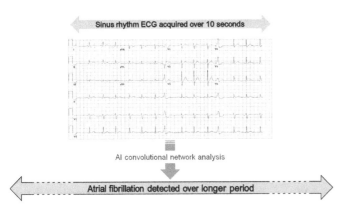

Fig. 2. A trained AI convolutional neural network may transform a standard spot ECG in sinus rhythm to a surrogate for prolonged rhythm monitoring for the detection of silent AF. (*Modified from* Siontis KC, Noseworthy PA, Attia ZI and Friedman PA. Artificial intelligence-enhanced electrocardiography in cardiovascular disease management. Nat Rev Cardiol. 2021; with permission).

an elderly patient with ESUS who had a high AI-ECG–derived probability of AF on an ECG preceding the ESUS event by 12 years.[19] Five years after the first stroke, the patient had a recurrent stroke and was clinically documented to have AF shortly thereafter, 17 years after the first ECG had indicated an elevated AF risk by AI analysis. An earlier intervention for thromboembolic risk reduction based on the results of AI-ECG analysis may have prevented her recurrent stroke. Furthermore, the diagnostic utility of AI-ECG for AF detection may be improved by AI analysis on serial ECGs that are acquired days, weeks, or months apart. We are currently testing the AF AI-ECG algorithm prospectively in the BEAGLE trial (NCT04208971) in which patients with a high AI-ECG score for AF and a high CHA2DS2VASc score (determined electronically via natural language processing [NLP]) are invited electronically to participate in prospective validation with a 30-day patch rhythm monitor for detection of incident AF. This trial highlights the promise of AI and electronic records in the real world. Patients are automatically identified for stroke risk via NLP chart review; automatically screened for silent AF via a stored normal sinus rhythm ECG using the AI screening of the ECG, and automatically invited to enroll in a study to prospectively detect AF, which will permit introduction of stroke prevention therapy.

Detection of Hypertrophic Cardiomyopathy

Although many patients with HCM have an abnormal ECG, there are no pathognomonic ECG changes in HCM. HCM can remain undiagnosed until symptoms develop or until cardiac imaging is performed for any reason. Using an established Mayo Clinic HCM cohort, we developed a CNN for the detection of HCM based on the 12-lead ECG and demonstrated an AUC of the CNN equal to 0.96 with sensitivity 87% and specificity 90%.[11] Noteworthy, the CNN model was able to reliably distinguish HCM from non-HCM LVH and was also able to detect HCM even from a seemingly normal ECG. Overall performance was best in younger patients (<40 years). Model performance using single-lead ECG data was similar to the 12-lead ECG performance. In separate work from another group of investigators, a different ML model was developed for the detection of HCM from the 12-lead ECG also with high accuracy (AUC of 0.91).[20] These algorithms may provide opportunities for targeted HCM screening in the future. In ongoing, preliminary work (yet unpublished), we are also exploring the potential of the HCM AI-ECG algorithm as a marker of treatment response in patients with HCM treated with targeted medical therapy. A home-based, single- or multi-lead ECG device with online connection to an AI-ECG analysis center may allow patients with HCM to continuously self-monitor their treatment response in the future.

RHYTHM DETERMINATION WITH WEARABLES

ML-powered, Internet-connected, direct-to-consumer wearables (watches, wristbands, textiles, smartphone-based applications) now offer real-time interpretation of biosignals, including those related to the cardiac rhythm, sleep patterns, fitness habits, and levels of blood oxygen, among others. Two approaches for rhythm determination have been largely used, including PPG and ECG recordings, as described previously. This section provides a framework for the evidence base of AI applications on automated PPG-based and ECG-based rhythm detection.

Pulse Photoplethysmography-Based Rhythm Detection

The Apple Heart Study is a landmark study in the wearable rhythm monitoring space both for its innovative design but also the important insights that it provides.[21] More than 400,000 participants were enrolled using electronic consent to passive PPG monitoring via their Apple Watch for irregular pulse detection suggestive of possible AF. Patients with possible AF detected via their smartwatch further underwent a confirmatory 7-day patch ECG monitoring. Similar to other tools using PPG, determination of pulse irregularity is performed by real-time automated analysis of heart rate variability tachograms collected once every 2 hours. A higher degree of dispersion of interpeak intervals correlates with a higher likelihood of pulse irregularity. However, the precise threshold of dispersion meeting criteria of irregularity and possible AF detection is proprietary and specific to this particular smartwatch technology. The user receives a notification for abnormal pulse detection if at least 5 of 6 consecutive tachograms within a 48-hour period are classified as irregular. In the Apple Heart Study, 0.52% of participants received at least 1 notification of possible AF over a median of 117 days. A small portion of these participants underwent 7-day rhythm monitoring and AF was detected in approximately one-third of them. In another large-scale, pragmatic assessment (MAFA II study), Guo and colleagues[22] investigated the effectiveness of a combination of passive and active AF screening using smart device-based PPG in a large Chinese population of approximately a quarter million participants with Huawei smartphones and PPG-capable devices. Of them, 0.23% received a possible AF notification. In turn, 87% had AF confirmed via various methods. These findings suggest that although mass screening of unselected populations is feasible with current technologies, the yield of PPG-based screening using a smart device may be low and with yet uncertain clinical impact. An important reason for this may be the young age and low risk profile of many smartwatch users. The clinical impact of smartwatch-based screening for AF is being investigated in the ongoing Heartline study (NCT04276441) in which participants older than 65 years without a history of AF are randomized to rhythm monitoring with an Apple Watch series 5 or later, versus routine care. Endpoints of interest include new diagnoses of AF, but also new anticoagulant prescriptions and major cardiovascular events, including stroke.[23]

Recently, Tison and colleagues[24] have reported on a deep neural network for the passive detection of AF based on the Apple Watch PPG technology. The investigators used heuristic pretraining in which the network approximates representations of the R-R interval without manual labeling of training data. Against a reference standard of AF diagnosed by 12-lead ECG in a validation cohort of patients undergoing cardioversion for AF, the AUC was 0.97, with corresponding sensitivity 98% and specificity 90%. Another group of investigators trained a CNN to detect AF in PPG waveforms from publicly available databases and validated the network in smartphone-acquired PPG recordings of high-risk patients for AF using expert cardiologist ECG interpretations as the reference standard.[25] The AUC of the CNN for AF detection was 0.997, with sensitivity and specificity equal to 95.2% and 99.0%, respectively, using a single 17-second PPG recording. Although these early results are encouraging, assessment of real-world performance will be essential given the multiple sources of noise and artifact found in daily life.

DL applications on PPG data collected by smartwatches may overcome the challenges of rule-based algorithms for the detection of possible AF. In particular, PPG recordings in active individuals are associated with noise contamination despite attempts for signal filtering and denoising, and are associated with a wide range of heart rate variability depending on the individual's day-to-day activity level. The more traditional rule-based algorithms currently available for real-time rhythm classification as studied in the Apple Heart Study and in the MAFA II study may be relatively inaccurate in distinguishing true signal from noise. In contrast, it appears possible to train DL neural network models to learn the characteristics and patterns of noise without the need for manual labeling. Indeed, a DL method using unsupervised transfer learning through convolutional denoising autoencoders was recently implemented successfully for the assessment of signal quality and real-time AF detection from wearable PPG devices.[26]

In addition to smartwatch-based PPG recordings, smartphone camera applications using contact-free facial or fingertip PPG recordings may also be able to analyze rhythm irregularities for AF detection. In a meta-analysis of 10 diagnostic performance studies, overall pooled sensitivity and specificity for AF detection was 94.2% and 95.8%, respectively.[27] However, the positive predictive value for detecting AF in an asymptomatic patients aged 65 years and older was between 19.3% and 37.5%, suggesting that such applications in asymptomatic individuals may generate a disproportionately high number of false positive results.

Electrocardiogram-Based Rhythm Detection

The accuracy of rhythm determination based on PPG may be limited by signal quality issues especially in active ambulatory patients.[24] In the WATCH-AF trial that compared the diagnostic

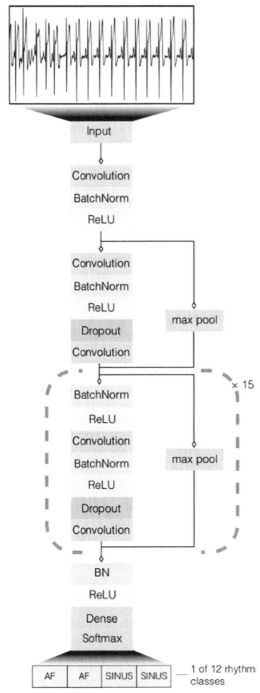

performance of a smartwatch-based PPG algorithm with physician's ECG diagnoses of AF, nearly 1 in 4 patients could not be included in analyses due to insufficient signal quality.[28] Newer software and hardware, including the new iterations of the Apple Watch, can perform ambulatory rhythm determination using electrophysiological signals (rather than PPG) obtained with one or more bipolar vectors.[29] Unlike the continuous passive rhythm detection from PPG signals, these applications currently require patient activation to record a rhythm strip. Using these signals, the application of DL approaches, particularly CNNs, has proven feasible and early results are promising for providing real-time, accurate automated feature discovery and rhythm classification.[29–31] In a notable example, Hannun and colleagues[29] developed a deep neural network to classify 12 rhythm classes, including artifact, using more than 90,000 single-lead ECGs from an ECG monitor patch (**Fig. 3**) (Zio monitor; iRhythm Technologies, Inc, San Francisco, CA). The network achieved an average AUC of 0.97 when validated against a testing dataset annotated by expert interpreters. Teplitzky and colleagues[30] also trained DL models for beat and rhythm classification from real-world single-lead recordings of the Body-Guardian monitor (Preventice Solutions, Rochester, MN) with high accuracy. F1 scores exceeded 70 for all 14 rhythm classes of interest, whereas for 5 of them the F1 scores exceeded 95, including for AF, ventricular tachycardia, ventricular bigeminy, ventricular trigeminy, and third-degree heart block.[30]

In a clinical validation study, Bumgarner and colleagues[32] tested whether a single-lead ECG recording obtained with the Kardia Band (AliveCor, Mountain View, CA), which was coupled with the Apple Watch could be used to distinguish AF from sinus rhythm in patients presenting for cardioversion. The determination of AF was based on traditional algorithmic approach measuring rhythm irregularity and absence of P wave rather than deep learning. Among interpretable recordings, AF was detected with 93% sensitivity and specificity 84%. The Kardia Band is no longer commercially available but has been replaced by the single-lead and 6-lead KardiaMobile devices that are FDA approved as home-based rhythm recording devices and are powered by deep-learning AI analytics for real-time rhythm classification.

Fig. 3. Deep Neural Network architecture for rhythm classification using a single-lead ECG monitor. The deep neural network consisted of 33 convolutional layers followed by a linear output layer into a softmax. The network accepts raw ECG data as input (sampled at 200 Hz, or 200 samples per second), and outputs a prediction of one out of 12 possible rhythm classes every 256 input samples. (*From* Hannun AY, Rajpurkar P, Haghpanahi M, Tison GH, Bourn C, Turakhia MP and Ng AY. Cardiologist-level arrhythmia detection and classification in ambulatory electrocardiograms using a deep neural network. Nat Med. 2019;25:65-69; with permission.)

Our group and others have recently reported the development of CNNs that are able to output fully automated comprehensive ECG interpretation with high fidelity using raw ECG data as the model input.[33,34] As we have previously demonstrated with CNNs trained for ECG-based detection of low ejection fraction and HCM, it is possible to fine-tune this AI-ECG interpretation software for implementation on single-lead recordings. We have also demonstrated the ability to determine the QT interval accurate with the addition of AI to a 2-channel smartphone-enabled ECG, potentially permitting point-of-care long QT screening.[35] This is becoming particularly important as the expanding popularity of wearable consumer-facing applications continues to increase the volume of signals that require interpretation. Such an approach may also facilitate the scalability of telehealth technologies through the availability of virtual core interpretation facilities with real-time, Internet-based input of large amounts of data and rapid result feedback. This type of infrastructure along with an understanding of the complex regulatory and privacy requirements are just now starting to emerge.[36,37]

DIGITAL PHENOTYPING OF ATRIAL FIBRILLATION

In patients with AF, ML applications on the standard ECG and on patient-obtained tracings have the potential to improve disease phenotyping and risk stratification, and help guide clinical decision-making. In a study using data from implanted cardiac devices in more than 3000 patients with AF, supervised machine-learning models, including random forest, CNN and L1 regularized logistic regression, were trained based on implanted device-recorded AF burden signatures to predict the risk of stroke.[38] All 3 ML models demonstrated superior performance for stroke prediction compared with the CHA2DS2-VASc score, the most widely used stroke-prediction scheme in practice.[39] Kaplan and colleagues[40] also demonstrated that AF duration as determined by implanted cardiac devices was a more powerful discriminator of stroke risk compared with the CHA2DS2-VASc score alone.

It has been postulated that a paradigm of intermittent anticoagulation for patients with paroxysmal AF guided by implanted device-based rhythm monitoring may be feasible. Early studies were underpowered to detect any significant clinical effects of such approaches.[41,42] However, in theory, AI models could be trained to use ECG

recordings and other physiologic signals/markers (eg, heart rate variability, frequency of ectopy, thoracic impedance changes, activity level changes) from implanted cardiac devices, or commercially available wearable ECG devices to predict impeding AF episodes. Patients could then receive a notification to alert them to self-administer a pill-in-pocket direct oral anticoagulant or even a pill-in-pocket antiarrhythmic agent. As an extension of this paradigm, beyond biometric signals such as the ECG, additional input data could be incorporated in multicomponent ML models that would be enriched with demographic, clinical, imaging, circulating biomarker data automatically retrievable from the electronic health record to predict short-term risk of arrhythmia or other adverse outcomes. These models can undergo continuous self-training with validation and calibration based on new clinical information and events (such as a new stroke event), such that after sufficient accumulation of experience they can provide precise estimations of risk to the clinician. The rhythm monitoring hardware, AI model infrastructure, and large clinical datasets are already available to develop such innovative paradigms that seemingly belong in the far future, but rigorous clinical investigation and validation are required.

SUMMARY

Electrical signals recorded from the body surface are rich in cardiac and noncardiac physiologic information that is useful for detecting silent or impending disease. AI can detect subtle, nonlinear, potentially interrelated signal perturbations to identify disease-specific patterns previously hidden in complex physiologic signals. This will accelerate the progress achieved in the arrhythmia monitoring space by improving the accuracy and efficiency of rhythm determination from electrophysiologic signals acquired by millions of people globally. In some cases, it may eliminate the need to monitor for and detect the actual arrhythmia by recognizing the physiologic changes leading up to the arrhythmia before the rhythm disturbance manifests. Demonstration of the real-world impact of AI-enabled arrhythmia monitoring on outcomes that are important to patients and other stakeholders, including the efficiency of telehealth care and greater independence from the traditional, resource intensive, face-to-face clinical care, will be required to drive demand for AI-integrated monitoring and to define its proper role in practice. Remaining challenges that need to be addressed for these applications to be more massively integrated into practice include the availability of widely accessible tools for low-cost implementation, the establishment of regulatory and legal frameworks for the transfer, storage, and analysis of data acquired by consumer-facing wearables without jeopardizing patient privacy, as well as the establishment of payment and reimbursement models for telehealth AI-enabled services. Despite these challenges, the application of AI to physiologic monitoring stands to enable the early detection and potential prevention of serious medical conditions, precise phenotyping of conditions previously grouped together, and ultimately improved human health.

CLINICS CARE POINTS

- Application of AI analysis to physiologic signals from the standard ECG and rhythm monitoring devices is feasible and increasingly integrated in clinical practice.

- In the near future, comprehensive cardiac phenotyping will be possible with the application of multiple AI-ECG algorithms on a single ECG.

- Integration of AI results from ECG and rhythm monitoring data in a patient's electronic health record is underway for use at the forefront of care.

- The impact of AI-ECG tools on the patient outcomes and cost-effectiveness of patient care is now beginning to be evaluated.

DISCLOSURE

Mayo Clinic, K.C.S., and P.A.F. have filed patents on AI-ECG algorithms discussed in this article.

REFERENCES

1. Attia ZI, Noseworthy PA, Lopez-Jimenez F, et al. An artificial intelligence-enabled ECG algorithm for the identification of patients with atrial fibrillation during sinus rhythm: a retrospective analysis of outcome prediction. Lancet 2019;394:861–7.

2. Levy AE, Biswas M, Weber R, et al. Applications of machine learning in decision analysis for dose management for dofetilide. PLoS One 2019;14: e0227324.

3. Gottesman O, Johansson F, Komorowski M, et al. Guidelines for reinforcement learning in healthcare. Nat Med 2019;25:16–8.

4. Krittanawong C, Johnson KW, Rosenson RS, et al. Deep learning for cardiovascular medicine: a practical primer. Eur Heart J 2019;40:2058–73.

5. Siontis KC, Yao X, Pirruccello JP, et al. How will machine learning inform the clinical care of atrial fibrillation? Circ Res 2020;127:155–69.

6. Deo RC. Machine learning in medicine. Circulation 2015;132:1920–30.

7. Arquilla K, Webb AK, Anderson AP. Textile electrocardiogram (ECG) electrodes for wearable health monitoring. Sensors (Basel) 2020;20:1013.

8. Krittanawong C, Rogers AJ, Johnson KW, et al. Integration of novel monitoring devices with machine learning technology for scalable cardiovascular management. Nat Rev Cardiol 2020;18(2):p75–91.

9. Pereira T, Tran N, Gadhoumi K, et al. Photoplethysmography based atrial fibrillation detection: a review. NPJ Digit Med 2020;3:3.

10. Attia ZI, Kapa S, Lopez-Jimenez F, et al. Screening for cardiac contractile dysfunction using an artificial intelligence-enabled electrocardiogram. Nat Med 2019;25:70–4.

11. Ko WY, Siontis KC, Attia ZI, et al. Detection of hypertrophic cardiomyopathy using a convolutional neural network-enabled electrocardiogram. J Am Coll Cardiol 2020;75:722–33.

12. Attia ZI, Friedman PA, Noseworthy PA, et al. Age and sex estimation using artificial intelligence from standard 12-lead ECGs. Circ-Arrhythmia Elec 2019;12: e007284.

13. Diez Benavente E, Jimenez-Lopez F, Attia Z, et al. Studying accelerated cardiovascular ageing in Russian adults through a novel deep-learning ECG biomarker [version 1; peer review: awaiting peer review]. Wellcome Open Res 2021;6:e007284.

14. Available at: https://www.fda.gov/media/137930/download. Accessed February 3, 2021.

15. Curry SJ, Krist AH, Owens DK, et al. Screening for atrial fibrillation with electrocardiography: US preventive services task force recommendation statement. JAMA 2018;320:478–84.

16. Hart RG, Sharma M, Mundl H, et al. Rivaroxaban for stroke prevention after embolic stroke of undetermined source. N Engl J Med 2018;378:2191–201.

17. Diener HC, Sacco RL, Easton JD, et al. Dabigatran for prevention of stroke after embolic stroke of undetermined source. N Engl J Med 2019;380: 1906–17.

18. Christopoulos G, Graff-Radford J, Lopez CL, et al. Artificial intelligence-electrocardiography to predict incident atrial fibrillation: a population-based study. Circ Arrhythm Electrophysiol 2020;13:e009355.

19. Kashou AH, Rabinstein AA, Attia IZ, et al. Recurrent cryptogenic stroke: a potential role for an artificial intelligence-enabled electrocardiogram? Heartrhythm Case Rep 2020;6:202–5.

20. Tison GH, Zhang J, Delling FN, et al. Automated and interpretable patient ECG profiles for disease detection, tracking, and discovery. Circ Cardiovasc Qual Outcomes 2019;12:e005289.

21. Perez MV, Mahaffey KW, Hedlin H, et al. Large-scale assessment of a smartwatch to identify atrial fibrillation. N Engl J Med 2019;381:1909–17.

22. Guo Y, Wang H, Zhang H, et al. Mobile photoplethysmographic technology to detect atrial fibrillation. J Am Coll Cardiol 2019;74:2365–75.

23. Heartline study. Available at: https://clinicaltrials.gov/ct2/show/NCT04276441. Accessed February 3, 2021.

24. Tison GH, Sanchez JM, Ballinger B, et al. Passive detection of atrial fibrillation using a commercially available smartwatch. JAMA Cardiol 2018;3:409–16.

25. Poh MZ, Poh YC, Chan PH, et al. Diagnostic assessment of a deep learning system for detecting atrial fibrillation in pulse waveforms. Heart 2018;104:1921–8.

26. Torres-Soto J, Ashley EA. Multi-task deep learning for cardiac rhythm detection in wearable devices. NPJ Digit Med 2020;3:116.

27. O'Sullivan JW, Grigg S, Crawford W, et al. Accuracy of smartphone camera applications for detecting atrial fibrillation: a systematic review and meta-analysis. JAMA Netw Open 2020;3:e202064.

28. Dorr M, Nohturfft V, Brasier N, et al. The WATCH AF trial: SmartWATCHes for detection of atrial fibrillation. JACC Clin Electrophysiol 2019;5:199–208.

29. Hannun AY, Rajpurkar P, Haghpanahi M, et al. Cardiologist-level arrhythmia detection and classification in ambulatory electrocardiograms using a deep neural network. Nat Med 2019;25:65–9.

30. Teplitzky BA, McRoberts M, Ghanbari H. Deep learning for comprehensive ECG annotation. Heart Rhythm 2020;17:881–8.

31. Xiong Z, Nash MP, Cheng E, et al. ECG signal classification for the detection of cardiac arrhythmias using a convolutional recurrent neural network. Physiol Meas 2018;39:094006.

32. Bumgarner JM, Lambert CT, Hussein AA, et al. Smartwatch algorithm for automated detection of atrial fibrillation. J Am Coll Cardiol 2018;71:2381–8.

33. Zhu H, Cheng C, Yin H, et al. Automatic multilabel electrocardiogram diagnosis of heart rhythm or conduction abnormalities with deep learning: a cohort study. Lancet Digit Health 2020;2:e348–57.

34. Kashou AH, Ko W-Y, Attia ZI, et al. A comprehensive artificial intelligence–enabled electrocardiogram interpretation program. Cardiovasc Digital Health J 2020;1:62–70.

35. Giudicessi JR, Schram M, Bos JM, et al. Artificial intelligence-enabled assessment of the heart rate corrected QT interval using a mobile electrocardiogram device. Circulation 2021;143(13):p.1274–86.

36. Tarakji KG, Silva J, Chen LY, et al. Digital health and the care of the patient with arrhythmia: what every electrophysiologist needs to Know. Circ Arrhythm Electrophysiol 2020;13:e007953.

37. The US Food and Drug Administration. US FDA artificial intelligence and machine learning discussion 2019. Available at: https://www.fda.gov/files/medical%20devices/published/US-FDA-Artificial-Intelligence-and-Machine-Learning-Discussion-Paper.pdf. Accessed February 3, 2021.

38. Han L, Askari M, Altman RB, et al. Atrial fibrillation burden signature and near-term prediction of stroke: a machine learning analysis. Circ Cardiovasc Qual Outcomes 2019;12:e005595.

39. Lip GY, Nieuwlaat R, Pisters R, et al. Refining clinical risk stratification for predicting stroke and thromboembolism in atrial fibrillation using a novel risk factor-based approach: the euro heart survey on atrial fibrillation. Chest 2010;137:263–72.

40. Kaplan RM, Koehler J, Ziegler PD, et al. Stroke risk as a function of atrial fibrillation duration and CHA2DS2-VASc score. Circulation 2019;140:1639–46.

41. Passman R, Leong-Sit P, Andrei AC, et al. Targeted anticoagulation for atrial fibrillation guided by continuous rhythm assessment with an insertable cardiac monitor: the rhythm evaluation for anticoagulation with continuous monitoring (REACT.COM) pilot study. J Cardiovasc Electrophysiol 2016;27:264–70.

42. Waks JW, Passman RS, Matos J, et al. Intermittent anticoagulation guided by continuous atrial fibrillation burden monitoring using dual-chamber pacemakers and implantable cardioverter-defibrillators: results from the Tailored Anticoagulation for Non-Continuous Atrial Fibrillation (TACTIC-AF) pilot study. Heart Rhythm 2018;15:1601–7.

43. Ribeiro AH, Ribeiro MH, Paixao GMM, et al. Automatic diagnosis of the 12-lead ECG using a deep neural network. Nat Commun 2020;11:1760.

44. Attia ZI, Kapa S, Yao XX, et al. Prospective validation of a deep learning electrocardiogram algorithm for the detection of left ventricular systolic dysfunction. J Cardiovasc Electrophysiol 2019;30:668–74.

45. Galloway CD, Valys AV, Shreibati JB, et al. Development and validation of a deep-learning model to screen for hyperkalemia from the electrocardiogram. JAMA Cardiol 2019;4:428–36.

46. Noseworthy PA, Attia ZI, Brewer LC, et al. Assessing and mitigating bias in medical artificial intelligence: the effects of race and ethnicity on a deep learning model for ECG analysis. Circ Arrhythm Electrophysiol 2020;13:e007988.

47. Adedinsewo D, Carter R, Attia IZ, et al. An artificial intelligence-enabled ECG algorithm to identify patients with left ventricular systolic dysfunction presenting to the emergency department with

dyspnea. Circ Arrhythm Electrophysiol 2020;13(8): e008437.

48. Raghunath S, Ulloa Cerna AE, Jing L, et al. Prediction of mortality from 12-lead electrocardiogram voltage data using a deep neural network. Nat Med 2020;26:886–91.

49. Chen TM, Huang CH, Shih ESC, et al. Detection and classification of cardiac arrhythmias by a challenge-best deep learning neural network model. iScience 2020;23:100886.

50. Feeny AK, Rickard J, Trulock KM, et al. Machine learning of 12-lead QRS waveforms to identify cardiac resynchronization therapy patients with differential outcomes. Circ Arrhythm Electrophysiol 2020;13:e008210.

Returning Cardiac Rhythm Data to Patients
Opportunities and Challenges

Ruth Masterson Creber, PhD, MSc, RN*,
Meghan Reading Turchioe, PhD, MPH, RN

KEYWORDS

- Atrial fibrillation • Cardiac electrophysiology • Cardiac implantable electronic devices
- Consumer electrocardiogram devices • Heart rhythm • Mobile health applications
- Remote monitoring • Visualization

KEY POINTS

- The impetus for sharing data comes from both a push from the federal government through the 21st Century Cures Act and the Heart Rhythm Society as well as a pull from patients to share patient health data (such as arrhythmia episodes, changes in health status, and device status) with more transparency.
- Reasons for returning patient health data include increasing transparency, deeper insights into personal health status, improved ability to schedule and manage follow-up care, and prevention of emergencies such as low battery or data transmission errors.
- Data can be returned using consumer applications and devices to monitor cardiac rhythm, including mobile health (mHealth) apps and consumer electrocardiogram devices.
- Three major challenges for returning patient information are patient comprehension of health data, management of patient–health care professional communication to reduce patient-level anxiety, and sustained patient engagement over time.
- Three recommendations for addressing challenges are to develop visualizations to support and aid comprehension of complex information, set clear goals and expectations with patients about data exchange, and develop patient-facing digital tools with participatory design methods including end-users to align features with their unique needs and preferences.

INTRODUCTION

Atrial fibrillation (AF) is highly prevalent, affecting an estimated 37 million people globally.[1] Its prevalence continues to climb dramatically; it is estimated that 12 million individuals in the United States alone will have AF by 2030.[2] AF is a complex chronic cardiac condition that requires routine self-management to reduce risks of stroke and mortality.[3–10] AF represents a major public health burden, accounting for more than 750,000 hospitalizations, 130,000 deaths, and $6 billion in costs each year.[2]

Timely detection of AF, initiation of thromboembolic prophylaxis, and often restoration of normal sinus rhythm are critical to improve disease management through medication and lifestyle adjustments and reduce negative health outcomes of AF, such as hospitalization, stroke, or death.[11,10] Timely detection also has the potential to improve quality of life and reduce the public health burden of AF.[11,12] The most common approaches for detecting and managing AF typically include brief windows of electrocardiogram (ECG) monitoring and 12-lead ECGs at prescheduled health visits.[13] These approaches are inadequate given the sporadic, unpredictable nature of arrhythmia, so AF often goes undetected and thus untreated.[11,13]

Division of Health Informatics, Weill Cornell Medicine, 425 E 61st St, Floor 3, New York, NY 10065, USA
* Corresponding author.
E-mail address: rmc2009@med.cornell.edu

Card Electrophysiol Clin 13 (2021) 555–567
https://doi.org/10.1016/j.ccep.2021.05.002
1877-9182/21/© 2021 Elsevier Inc. All rights reserved.

Across health care sectors, digital health tools are transforming patient access to their health data and empowering them to assume a more central role in detecting symptoms and self-managing their condition. In cardiology, novel digital cardiac devices represent a convergence between health care and emerging digital technologies and include tools intended for health care providers, patients, or both. In the field of cardiac electrophysiology, digital health tools for AF fall into 4 primary categories: *cardiac implantable electronic devices (CIEDs)*, *consumer ECG devices*, *mobile health applications (mHealth apps)*, and *medical-grade telemetry monitors*. The 2019 clinical guidelines for managing patients with AF include recommendations for using CIEDs to detect silent AF in patients with cryptogenic stroke over age 40.[14] The guidelines also acknowledge the potential role that consumer ECG devices and mHealth apps have for screening and timely detection of arrhythmias, including silent AF.

The growth of consumer ECG devices and mHealth apps represents novel opportunities to assist AF patients with AF self-management. Consumer ECG devices such as the AliveCor device allow individuals with AF to easily record and transmit an ECG to their health care provider for review using a device that is interoperable with both iOS and Android smartphones. The AliveCor algorithm in the mHealth app that accompanies the device attempts to identify arrhythmias such as AF.[15] The SEARCH-AF study found that using this technology in community settings was both cost-effective and feasible.[16] The integration of ECG technology with mHealth apps can support population screening and timely detection of AF.

The Apple Watch is another example of a consumer ECG device that enables individuals to record a single-lead ECG in an easy, accurate, and timely manner.[17] As these devices improve in precision, they also facilitate earlier diagnosis of AF recurrence[18] and population screening for AF among currently undiagnosed (estimated to be 13%)[19] and asymptomatic patients with AF.

From the patient perspective, individuals with AF perceive a need for ECG mHealth technology. In a recent survey, most individuals living with a cardiac condition, such as AF, reported a need for technology-based support to increase health knowledge, decrease travel and accessibility restraints, and better use peer support.[20] Given the increased accessibility of digital health tools for population screening and timely detection and interest among patients to use these devices, there are significant opportunities and challenges for the future of patient-facing heart rhythm data.

THE HISTORY AND EVOLUTION OF PATIENT-FACING DATA IN ELECTROPHYSIOLOGY

Whereas using medical and consumer technologies to monitor patients with a range of chronic conditions has become increasingly popular in recent years,[21] cardiac electrophysiology has been at the forefront of remote patient monitoring for decades. However, since its introduction in the 1970s, remote monitoring has primarily been used to inform health care providers about patients' cardiac rhythm and function outside of clinical settings and guide medical decision-making.

The important role of patients in ensuring continued device communication in remote monitoring, troubleshooting device problems, attending follow-up appointments for interrogation, and understanding what to do in an emergency because of delays in transmission has been acknowledged in recent years. This has led to expert recommendations from the Heart Rhythm Society (HRS) to educate patients about remote monitoring and their unique responsibilities in the process.[22] As the trend of engaging patients in remote monitoring has continued to gain popularity, and technologies and platforms to monitor cardiac rhythm and share health data electronically have become increasingly available to patients, the interest in and efforts to return cardiac rhythm data and other data about health status to patients have grown. While using digital health tools to monitor and share cardiac rhythm data with patients has been conducted mostly for AF screening and management, the return of these data may also benefit patients with many other arrhythmias in the future.[22]

THE RATIONALE FOR RETURNING CARDIAC RHYTHM DATA TO PATIENTS

The impetus for returning cardiac rhythm data has experienced both a *"push"* from the federal government and professional societies and a *"pull"* from patients to share CIED data with greater transparency about their health information. Together these forces support a strong rationale for returning CIED data to patients. The Office of the National Coordinator for Health Information Technology (ONC), a branch of the Department of Health and Human Services, released the final rule from the 21st Century Cures Act, effective June 2020.[23] The new provisions in the final rule support interoperability and support access, exchange, and use of electronic health information by patients. This ruling is consistent with expert recommendations from the HRS to support interoperability of data from CIEDs.[24]

Currently, when patients receive any information about their CIEDs, it is typically limited to device status indicators (such as battery status and functioning of the mobile communicator).[25] Patients report that they would like to receive information about arrhythmia episodes, changes in health status over time, and more routine and detailed information about their device status and functioning.[25] Increasing transparency by providing access to their health information gives patients insight and more control over their care, including attending follow-up appointments for interrogation and preventing emergencies by being more prepared for events such as a low battery or other errors with data transmission.

The primary reasons for returning data to patients include the improved ability for patients to manage their health for both primary and secondary disease prevention as well as increased patient satisfaction. Studies of digital health information exchange from other domains have demonstrated positive health outcomes when patients have access to their health information.[26,27] Patients report an improved understanding of their disease and the factors contributing to it because they can collect and visualize their data more efficiently with digital technologies.[28,29] Patients also report that remote monitoring is acceptable, convenient, and associated with good quality of life.[30] This is critical because patient satisfaction and acceptance of remote follow-up are critical for successfully implementing remote monitoring.[30] Furthermore, the latest thinking from the digital health and research communities at large is that there is an ethical imperative to return these data to patients as the original source of the data and the key stakeholders in the care delivery process.[31,32]

In conclusion, the combination of the push from the ONC final rule and the HRS that represents electrophysiologists, as well as the pull from patients who want access to their health information, means that medical device companies and health care systems alike are reexamining existing models of remote patient monitoring and moving toward returning relevant cardiac health data to patients.[25]

AVENUES FOR RETURNING PATIENT DATA
Consumer Applications and Devices to Monitor Cardiac Rhythm

Digital health tools that are directly available to consumers are dramatically changing the health technology landscape across every discipline. Cardiology is no exception; consumer applications and devices offer patients the greatest access to their cardiac rhythm data and other relevant data about health compared with other technologies that collect or contain cardiac rhythm data. These devices allow patients to record and directly view cardiac information without requiring a health care professional to initiate or mediate data access. In this way, these devices act as a "window" into one's cardiac rhythm that is not often available to them. The 2 main areas of growth are in *mHealth apps,* which leverage native features and functionalities of the phone to monitor health, and other *consumer ECG devices*, which explicitly monitor cardiac rhythm.

mHealth apps may include functionalities to record, view, and share health data. They may also leverage the phone in these functionalities—most notably, they can create photoplethysmography (PPG) waveforms by using the light-emitting diode (LED) flash from a smartphone camera to detect changes in tissue blood volume in a user's finger.[33] An example of an mHealth app available to consumers for PPG waveform monitoring is the Qardio app, shown in **Fig. 1**. Several recent systematic reviews have noted an increasing number of applications being developed for AF, many of which include PPG waveform monitoring as their primary functionality.[34–36] These apps may also support medication adherence and symptom monitoring, motivate positive lifestyle behaviors, and provide relevant patient education.

mHealth apps offer the unique advantages of being free or low cost and leverage smartphone technology that 81% of Americans[37] and over 5 billion adults worldwide[38] already own. However, because cardiac rhythm monitoring is a functionality that can be supported with the technology but is not the sole or explicit purpose of it, the accuracy of mHealth apps to monitor cardiac rhythm is not as high as is it for *consumer ECG devices* explicitly designed for this purpose. Some consumer devices, such as the Apple Watch, have numerous functionalities and applications but have been engineered to allow users to directly measure and store their cardiac rate and rhythm data. Others, such as AliveCor's Kardia device, are simply hardware that directly records cardiac rate and rhythm but communicates with an mHealth app to visualize the rhythm to users and allow data to be stored and shared.

The inclusion of the cardiac rhythm monitoring feature in newer generations of the Apple Watch has generated much excitement because of its popularity and widespread adoption. The Apple Watch uses PPG technology to monitor pulse rate over time and contains an algorithm that can automatically identify irregular waveforms as a possible sign of AF.[39] The incorporation of this

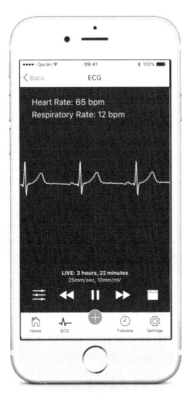

Fig. 1. The freely available Qardio provides PPG waveform monitoring to consumers.

technology into the popular consumer device has already been leveraged for population screening efforts on an unprecedented scale. The Apple Heart Study is likely the most dramatic example of this; in this study, the authors enrolled nearly 420,000 individuals over 8 months to use the Apple Watch for cardiac rhythm screening.[40] For those participants receiving irregular rhythm alerts, more intensive monitoring and cardiologist follow-up were initiated to confirm a diagnosis of AF.

Another device that has been available to patients for longer (it was first approved by the Food and Drug Administration in 2012) is the Kardia device made by AliveCor.[41] The device is a piece of lightweight hardware that attaches or can be placed next to a smartphone or tablet. The user places their fingertips on the device to record a 30 s single-lead (lead II) ECG. Using Wi-Fi or cellular network transmission, the device communicates with a Kardia smartphone application. In this application, users can view their ECGs as they record them, review prior ECGs, and share ECGs. Furthermore, the application employs a proprietary algorithm to detect AF. Research has shown that the ECG tracing is highly sensitive (100%) and specific (94%), but the algorithm

interpreting the ECG is somewhat less accurate (sensitivity: 55%–70%, specificity: 60%–69%).[42] Studies have found that patients find AliveCor easy to use.[43,44].

In addition, several mHealth apps do not directly measure cardiac rhythm but nonetheless collect and return valuable information to patients with arrhythmias. These applications are focused more generally on self-management and symptom monitoring and may be beneficial to patients with chronic arrhythmias such as AF. For example, several applications are designed to allow patients to track symptoms over time, visualize their data, and uncover trends that may help them better understand their symptoms. One example is the Symple application (https://www.sympleapp.com/), which allows users to track a wide range of symptoms and includes sophisticated visualizations of longitudinal symptom data (**Fig. 2**). Another example is the Medly application (https://medly.ca/), which allows patients to record daily weight, blood pressure, heart rate, and symptoms. It includes an algorithm that generates personalized self-care messages (eg, adjust diuretic medications) and sends real-time alerts to health care providers as needed. This application is currently being evaluated in the Medly-AID trial, a randomized, controlled trial in Canada.[45]

Patient-Facing Applications with Cardiac Implantable Electronic Devices

Some CIEDs come with patient portals or other mechanisms that show patients information about their CIEDs. The implications for returning data from CIEDs are distinct from other consumer technologies such as mHealth apps and consumer ECG devices. CIEDs are implantable, and thus, access to cardiac rhythm data requires more technical steps, as devices may need to be interrogated or transmissions may only be available to health care providers and not the patient. In contrast, many consumer ECG devices and mHealth apps make cardiac rhythm data immediately viewable, offering opportunities for population-level screening of arrhythmias in addition to ongoing monitoring and management.[46]

Therefore, attention has focused on providing timely access to device data along with nontechnical summaries of device functionality and relevant clinical implications.[47] Most often, this information includes device battery status and functioning of the communicator. Recently there has been increased interest in sharing information about cardiac events and other health data collected with these devices. For example, the

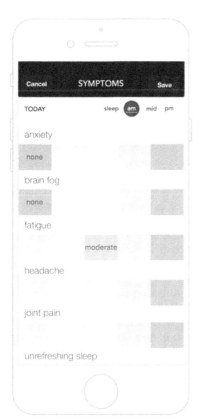

Fig. 2. The freely available Symple application allows users to track multiple symptoms and visualize longitudinal trends.

USC Center for Body Computing has developed a patient-facing, device-agnostic mHealth app for patients to visualize complex cardiac rhythm data in simplified ways, communicate with health care providers, and learn more about their arrhythmia.[48,49]

Inpatient Portals

Transparent access to personal health information has been championed for hospitalized patients to increase transparency and engage vulnerable patients with their health information in real-time.[50,51] Providing patient access to health information through a patient portal while in the hospital is termed an *inpatient portal*. Inpatient portals include access to medications being administered, short videos explaining the purpose of each medication as well as potential side effects, links to comprehensive medication information from MedlinePlus, documented allergies, diagnostic test orders and results, current documented diet, and vital signs and weight.[50] Access has also been hypothesized to improve patient activation, safety, and satisfaction with hospitals and health care providers.[52–59] The results of a randomized clinical trial among patients with heart failure did not result in improved patient activation, but it was associated with patients looking up health information online and a lower 30-day hospital readmission rate without increasing the burden on health care professionals and without a negative impact on direct health care delivery.[50] Overall, this study supports the growing body of evidence supporting transparent access to health information.

OPPORTUNITIES TO IMPROVE OUTCOMES THROUGH PATIENT-FACING DATA
Screening for Atrial Fibrillation

A significant opportunity exists to screen for arrhythmias using mHealth apps and consumer ECG devices. Many of these tools leverage PPG, which involves using light-based sensors to detect changes in tissue blood volume that result from peripheral pulses to create pulse waveforms. The LED flash from a smartphone camera can create PPG waveforms. As a result, smartphones can be used to record PPG waveforms; this creates a significant potential to monitor for arrhythmias, particularly AF, on a population level.[13] The fact that many mHealth apps that use PPG technology are freely available to patients improves their adoption and use by a wide range of individuals, including those who may lack the financial resources to use more expensive technologies for rhythm monitoring. For example, in a recent study, 12,000 individuals were screened for AF over 7 days using PPG, and 136 individuals (1%) screened positive for AF and then received a confirmatory clinical diagnosis of AF.[60]

However, a recent app review found the reviewed apps had wide variability in quality, functionality, and adherence to self-management behaviors.[36] Moreover, several studies have reported wide variability in the positive predictive values of these technologies for population screening, which suggests their performance may still vary among populations.[61–64] PPG waveforms are also prone to false-positive findings because they cannot distinguish among AF, atrial or ventricular premature contractions, and variable atrioventricular conduction (atrioventricular block).[60] Ultimately, patient and provider education must focus on the strengths and limitations of PPG waveforms for AF screening. These technologies should be used for screening but not confirmation of a diagnosis of a heart rhythm disorder; a 12-lead ECG or other guideline-recommended monitoring technology is still clinically necessary for diagnosis.

Self-Management and Self-Monitoring of Disease

AF is quite difficult to manage even with medication, lifestyle changes, and interventional procedures, such as ablations or the placement of internal monitors.[51,52] Even after procedures to restore normal sinus rhythm, AF recurrence is high. For example, the CABANA trial recently evaluated over 2200 symptomatic patients undergoing ablation and found that AF recurred in 50% of cases, and 17% needed a repeat ablation.[58]

Lifestyle-related risk factors for AF include stress, obesity, high cholesterol, poor nutrition, low exercise, hypertension, and smoking. The "iPhone Helping Evaluate Atrial Fibrillation Rhythm through Technology" (iHEART) trial is an example of a randomized control trial designed to support the prevention of AF recurrence and behavioral lifestyle interventions, including medication adherence, increased exercise, weight control, and a healthy diet.[44] Participants were given access to AliveCor and behavior-altering text messages centered on the American Heart Association's Life's Simple 7 educational materials and sent to patients with AF risk factors 3 times per week in English or Spanish.

Overall, the relationship between AF episodes and symptoms is complex and not well understood.[65–67] The reasons why some patients experience a heavy burden of symptoms but not a heavy AF burden, or the converse, is poorly understood.[65,66] Nonetheless, symptoms affect quality of life and are a primary indicator for ablation. Monitoring and managing symptoms is a critical aspect of AF management that can be facilitated with digital health tools. Common AF symptoms include physical and psychological symptoms, such as dyspnea, chest pain, fatigue, anxiety, and palpitations.[65] For many patients with AF, symptoms limit daily functioning and affect their quality of life.[67] Furthermore, patients have expressed a desire to better understand the relationship between their AF symptoms and cardiac rhythm.[25,68] Therefore, appropriate management of AF symptoms can improve quality of life and mitigate psychological distress.

Despite the clear need for increased symptom management in AF, the symptom tracking and visualization functionality in mHealth apps or consumer ECG devices for AF are still in their nascent stages.[36] Future technology should offer functionality that allows patients to track a range of physical and psychological symptoms, correlate symptoms with cardiac rhythm, lifestyle changes, and various therapies (medications, catheter ablation), and generate insights about strategies for improved management.[68]

Shared Decision-Making

Shared decision-making (SDM) is the process of discussing the risks and benefits of treatment options in the context of a patient's values, expectations, and preferences with the goal of selecting a treatment that aligns with these priorities.[69] SDM is an increasingly important and common practice that involves presenting health data to patients. SDM has been encouraged for many use cases in electrophysiology and even mandated by the Centers for Medicare and Medicaid Services in specific cases, such as in anticoagulation decisions for AF patients with high stroke risk.[35]

A central component of the SDM process is the use of decision aids. These are tools that present information about risks and benefits to improve patient knowledge, engagement, and satisfaction in the process.[70] Traditionally, decision aids have been paper-based pamphlets or educational materials that can be easily disseminated in clinical practices and other health care settings. Recently, many web-based decision aids have also been developed; these are often interactive, allowing the patient to specify details about themselves (demographics, medical history) and preferences for treatment so that the system can tailor the way information is displayed. Example—mayo. Drawbacks = access. Regardless of the medium, information visualization is frequently incorporated to support comprehension. For example, several visualization-based decision aids aimed at helping patients choose the right anticoagulant for stroke prevention in AF have been developed;[71–75] one example is shown in **Fig. 3**.

CHALLENGES AND RECOMMENDATIONS

Returning data to patients is still in its nascent stages, with several key questions remaining unanswered. Below we highlight 3 major challenges in the field to date and offer recommendations to address these challenges.

Challenges	Recommendations
(1) Comprehension of information	Develop visualizations to support and aid comprehension of complex information.
(2) Managing patient–health care professional communication to	Provide patient education and support, set clear goals and

(continued on next page)

CHA2DS2-VASc score of 3
HEMORR2HAGES score of 3

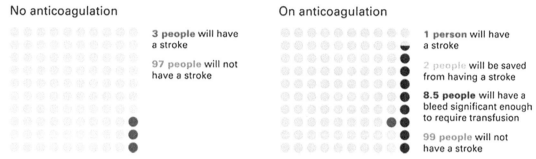

No anticoagulation

3 **people** will have a stroke

97 **people** will not have a stroke

On anticoagulation

1 **person** will have a stroke

2 people will be saved from having a stroke

8.5 people will have a bleed significant enough to require transfusion

99 people will not have a stroke

Fig. 3. Pictogram showing the annual stroke risk of a patient with atrial fibrillation and a CHADS2 score of 3. (*From* Seaburg L, Hess E, Coylewright M, Ting H, McLeod C, Montori V. Shared Decision Making in Atrial Fibrillation. Circulation. 2014;129(6):704-710. https://doi.org/10.1161/circulationaha.113.004498; with permission.)

(continued)	
Challenges	**Recommendations**
reduce patient-level anxiety	expectations around data exchange, consult stakeholders when establishing goals and expectations for a specific practice or organization.
(3) Sustaining patient engagement	Develop patient-facing digital health tools through participatory design with end-users to align features with unique needs and preferences.

Comprehension of Complex Informational from Remote Monitoring Tools

A significant challenge for the return of remote monitoring patient information is the exponential quantity of data that patients need to sort, interpret, and act on for the information to be relevant and useful. A significant barrier is low graph literacy that varies by education level and socioeconomic status.[76] In the United States, at least one-third of adults cannot correctly interpret graphs.[77] This is problematic because the majority of cardiac health information is returned to patients as line graphs.[78]

In the context of the challenge of comprehension, information visualizations are a promising solution to support patients in interpreting their health information.[79–81] Visualizations support cognitive processing by leveraging the human potential to perceive differences in the sizes, shapes, colors, and spatial positions of objects and give meaning to those differences.[82] Visualizations are particularly meaningful because they can support comprehension of information without relying on high literacy or numeracy skills. Colors can facilitate interpretation instead of text.[81] Real-time changes to visualizations are also easier to deliver when they are integrated into digital technologies.[79] Importantly, patients interpret complex visualizations from a different mental model than health care professionals who have advanced statistical and medical knowledge.[83,84]

Displaying raw results without interpretation or contextualization is at best ineffective[50,85] and at worst perpetuates *intervention-generated inequity*,[86] a phenomenon whereby well-intentioned interventions worsen existing health disparities rather than reduce them[50,85–89] and result in miscommunication.[90] Appropriate use of visualizations for returning patient information is needed to ensure that patients can understand, and when appropriate, act on health data in a safe and effective manner.[78]

An example of an application of visualization of complex cardiac data from implantable devices is found in a participatory design study by Ahmed and colleagues (**Fig. 4**).[91–93] Participatory design approaches are an important method to ensure that visualizations are acceptable to patients. In this work, the authors have conducted participatory design to create a dashboard displaying complex data from cardiac resynchronization therapy devices. Patients reported wanting to visualize a range of data elements, including daily pacing reports, symptoms, and health tips, in addition to device functioning (battery life and recorded events).[94]

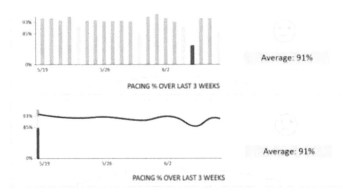

Fig. 4. An example patient-facing visualization of complex cardiac data from implantable devices published by Ahmed and colleagues. (*From* Ahmed R, Toscos T, Rohani Ghahari R et al. Visualization of Cardiac Implantable Electronic Device Data for Older Adults Using Participatory Design. Appl Clin Inform. 2019;10(04):707-718. https://doi.org/10.1055/s-0039-1695794; with permission.)

Managing Patient–Health Care Professional Communication to Reduce Patient-Level Anxiety About Patient Health Information

The possibility of a cardiac arrhythmia recurring, often with little to no warning, causes many patients with cardiac rhythm disorders to develop symptoms of anxiety.[95] For example, in the recent iHEART trial, over 30% of the 171 adults with AF enrolled in the trial reported clinically significant anxiety.[96] Furthermore, this study found that the severity of anxiety was associated with the severity of AF. In a separate qualitative study with iHEART trial participants, anxiety was commonly reported as both a reason for using digital technology (specifically, the AliveCor Kardia device), and a reason for discontinuing use.[68] Specifically, some participants reported that the ability to view their heart rhythm ameliorated questions about their cardiac rhythm, particularly if they did not typically experience symptomatic AF. Other patients and many providers reported that viewing their cardiac rhythm data so frequently caused them to focus even more on their rhythm, which increased anxiety and ultimately proved unhelpful to the patient.

As a result of this anxiety, the patient's natural reaction is to reach out to providers to explain their data and ameliorate concerns. However, this creates many workflow and logistical challenges. Current clinical workflows are not designed to accommodate patients reaching out about their health data, and critically important questions about reimbursement, time, staffing, roles, and scope of practice have yet to be fully answered.[29] Additionally, it may be difficult for providers to appraise the quality of health data patients collect using consumer devices; this relates to variability in both patient skills in collecting and recording health measurements and the quality of the technologies being used.[27] Privacy and confidentiality regulations around patient data (eg, Health Insurance Portability and Accountability Act, or HIPAA) also complicate these interactions. Patients and developers of different consumer technologies alike may not fully understand or comply with these regulations.[97] Furthermore, any health data patients may want to share can rarely be integrated into the EHR.[98] While a lack of EHR integration limits the ability of providers to review and respond to these health data, efforts to advance EHR integration are complicated by interoperability requirements and concerns about data quality and security.

The literature suggests that certain basic practices may be beneficial in clinical practice to improve expectations and communication about health data and reduce patient anxiety. These include providing education and support for patients to correctly collect and interpret health data and setting clear goals and expectations around data exchange, including establishing routines for data sharing, expected timeframes for responses about data, and instructions on what to do in an emergency.[21] However, several studies also note that goals and expectations need to be tailored to the exact clinical use case; therefore, organizations seeking to return health data to patients should carefully consider a range of stakeholder perspectives, including different types of health care providers and patients, when creating policies and procedures for exchanging health data.

Sustaining Patient Engagement

However, both within and beyond cardiology contexts, sustained engagement with digital health tools remains one of the most significant barriers to their clinical utility. Studies measuring self-monitoring over an extended period show that many patients using mHealth for self-monitoring discontinue use within 3 to 6 months of initiation, suggesting that patients are not engaged in the process for a sustained period.[99–101]

Little is known about personalized approaches to improve sustained engagement. Much of the existing literature on user engagement focuses on strategies to improve initial uptake rather than sustained engagement. Many have attempted to bolster sustained engagement by including certain mHealth features, such as gamification and incentives, but have generally been unsuccessful.[102,103] A promising alternative approach is to design technologies based on individual user characteristics that may predict sustained engagement. Previous studies have demonstrated that individual characteristics, such as age and disease status, affect sustained engagement with mHealth.[101,104,105] This is supported by focus group findings suggesting that control over mHealth features, the context provided with health data, and the data shared with health care providers would improve sustained engagement.[106,107] Recent studies also suggest that intrinsic motivation to manage health plays a role in engagement with these technologies.[108,109] These reported factors demonstrate the need for mHealth technologies to be personalized.

The length of time that mHealth users must sustain engagement with the technology is prespecified depending on the ultimate goal of use. The goal of these technologies is to better detect and treat cardiac arrhythmias in a timelier manner.[13] For paroxysmal arrhythmias including AF, longitudinal data collection is often more valuable than brief, discrete periods of monitoring because of the spontaneous and unpredictable nature of arrhythmia episodes. However, longitudinal data collection is only possible if patients remain engaged with self-monitoring for a sustained period. When captured longitudinally, these data can be shared with health care providers to diagnose, treat, and manage these conditions more quickly and efficiently.[11,13]

A critical question for future research surrounding consumer ECG devices, and mHealth apps specifically, is what length of time and what intensity of engagement are appropriate and clinically beneficial. While AF burden can automatically be quantified using CIEDs, it cannot be quantified using most consumer ECG devices or mHealth apps, as these do not provide continuous monitoring. Thus, questions of the appropriate frequency and duration of use for detecting and monitoring AF are of paramount importance for their clinical utility. Although previous work has identified the shortest periods with the highest diagnostic yield for CIEDs and medical-grade wearable devices, such as the Zio Patch, this question has yet to be explored for digital health tools.[110–112]

CLINICS CARE POINTS

- Visual aids, including graphics and data visualizations, should be used when returning personal health data to patients from remote monitoring tools to improve comprehension.
- Conversations with patients should occur before initiating remote monitoring to provide education and set clear expectations about exchanging, reviewing, and responding to remote monitoring data.
- Clinicians should advocate for clear policies at their health institutions about exchanging and interacting with patients about their remote monitoring data.

DISCLOSURE

RMC is supported by NIH/NINR (R00NR016275) & NIH/NHLBI (R01HL152021), and MRT is supported by NIH/NINR K99NR019124.

REFERENCES

1. Lippi G, Sanchis-Gomar F, Cervellin G. Global epidemiology of atrial fibrillation: an increasing epidemic and public health challenge. Int J Stroke 2020. 1747493019897870.
2. CDC. Atrial fibrillation fact sheet. 2020. Available at: http://www.cdc.gov/dhdsp/data_statistics/fact_sheets/fs_atrial_fibrillation.htm. Accessed November 20, 2020.
3. Patel NJ, Atti V, Mitrani RD, et al. Global rising trends of atrial fibrillation: a major public health concern. Heart 2018;104(24):1989–90.
4. Chugh SS, Havmoeller R, Narayanan K, et al. Worldwide epidemiology of atrial fibrillation: a global burden of disease 2010 study. Circulation 2014;129(8):837–47.
5. Sultan A, Lüker J, Andresen D, et al. Predictors of atrial fibrillation recurrence after catheter ablation: data from the German ablation registry. Sci Rep 2017;7(1):16678.
6. Verma A, Jiang C-Y, Betts TR, et al. Approaches to catheter ablation for persistent atrial fibrillation. N Engl J Med 2015;372(19):1812–22.

7. Members WC, Writing Committee Members, Fuster V, et al. ACC/AHA/ESC 2006 guidelines for the management of patients with atrial fibrillation: full text: a report of the American College of cardiology/American heart association task force on practice guidelines and the European society of cardiology committee for practice guidelines (Writing Committee to Revise the 2001 guidelines for the management of patients with atrial fibrillation) developed in collaboration with the European heart rhythm association and the heart rhythm society. Europace 2006;8(9):651–745.

8. Chugh SS, Blackshear JL, Shen WK, et al. Epidemiology and natural history of atrial fibrillation: clinical implications. J Am Coll Cardiol 2001;37(2):371–8.

9. Zhang L, Gallagher R, Neubeck L. Health-related quality of life in atrial fibrillation patients over 65 years: a review. Eur J Prev Cardiol 2015;22(8):987–1002.

10. Kochhäuser S, Joza J, Essebag V, et al. The impact of duration of atrial fibrillation recurrences on measures of health-related quality of life and symptoms. Pacing Clin Electrophysiol 2016;39(2):166–72.

11. Olgun Kucuk H, Kucuk U, Yalcin M, et al. Time to use mobile health devices to diagnose paroxysmal atrial fibrillation. Int J Cardiol 2015. https://doi.org/10.1016/j.ijcard.2015.10.159.

12. Steinhubl SR, Topol EJ. Moving from digitalization to digitization in cardiovascular care: why is it important, and what could it mean for patients and providers? J Am Coll Cardiol 2015;66(13):1489–96.

13. Turakhia MP, Kaiser DW. Transforming the care of atrial fibrillation with mobile health. J Interv Card Electrophysiol 2016;47(1):45–50.

14. January CT, Wann LS, Calkins H, et al. 2019 AHA/ACC/HRS focused update of the 2014 AHA/ACC/HRS guideline for the management of patients with atrial fibrillation: a report of the American College of cardiology/American heart association Task force on clinical practice guidelines and the heart rhythm society. J Am Coll Cardiol 2019;74(1):104–32.

15. Steinhubl SR, Mehta RR, Ebner GS, et al. Rationale and design of a home-based trial using wearable sensors to detect asymptomatic atrial fibrillation in a targeted population: the mHealth Screening to Prevent Strokes (mSToPS) trial. Am Heart J 2016;175:77–85.

16. Lowres N, Neubeck L, Salkeld G, et al. Feasibility and cost-effectiveness of stroke prevention through community screening for atrial fibrillation using iPhone ECG in pharmacies. Thromb Haemost 2014;111(06):1167–76.

17. Wasserlauf J, You C, Patel R, et al. Smartwatch performance for the detection and quantification of atrial fibrillation. Circ Arrhythm Electrophysiol 2019;12(6):e006834.

18. Goldenthal IL, Sciacca RR, Riga T, et al. Recurrent atrial fibrillation/flutter detection after ablation or cardioversion using the AliveCor KardiaMobile device: iHEART results. J Cardiovasc Electrophysiol 2019;30(11):2220–8.

19. Turakhia MP, Shafrin J, Bognar K, et al. Estimated prevalence of undiagnosed atrial fibrillation in the United States. PLoS One 2018;13(4):e0195088.

20. Disler RT, Inglis SC, Newton PJ, et al. Perspectives of online health information and support in chronic disease respiratory disease: focus group study. In: A34. Influence of behavioral and psychosocial factors in health outcomes. American Thoracic Society International Conference Abstracts. American Thoracic Society; 2015. p. A1386. Available at: https://www.atsjournals.org/doi/abs/10.1164/ajrccm-conference.2015.191.1_MeetingAbstracts.A1386.

21. Reading MJ, Merrill JA. Converging and diverging needs between patients and providers who are collecting and using patient-generated health data: an integrative review. J Am Med Inform Assoc Published Online 2018. https://doi.org/10.1093/jamia/ocy006.

22. Slotwiner D, Varma N, Akar JG, et al. HRS Expert Consensus Statement on remote interrogation and monitoring for cardiovascular implantable electronic devices. Heart Rhythm 2015;12(7):e69–100.

23. Health and Human Services Department. 21st Century Cures act: interoperability, information blocking, and the ONC health IT certification program. Fed Regist 2020;85:25642–961.

24. Slotwiner DJ, Abraham RL, Al-Khatib SM, et al. HRS White Paper on interoperability of data from cardiac implantable electronic devices (CIEDs). Heart Rhythm 2019;16(9):e107–27.

25. Slotwiner DJ, Tarakji KG, Al-Khatib SM, et al. Transparent sharing of digital health data: a call to action. Heart Rhythm 2019;16(9):e95–106.

26. Arsoniadis EG, Tambyraja R, Khairat S, et al. Characterizing patient-generated clinical data and associated implications for electronic health records. Stud Health Technol Inform 2015;216:158–62.

27. Lavallee DC, Chenok KE, Love RM, et al. Incorporating patient-reported outcomes into health care to engage patients and enhance care. Health Aff 2016;35(4):575–82.

28. Chung CF, Dew K, Cole A, et al. Boundary negotiating artifacts in personal informatics: patient-provider collaboration with patient-generated data. ACM 2016;770–86.

29. Howie L, Hirsch B, Locklear T, et al. Assessing the value of patient-generated data to comparative effectiveness research. Health Aff 2014;33(7):1220–8.

30. Zeitler EP, Piccini JP. Remote monitoring of cardiac implantable electronic devices (CIED). Trends Cardiovasc Med 2016;26(6):568–77.

31. Ballantyne A. How should we think about clinical data ownership? J Med Ethics 2020;46(5):289–94.

32. Schickhardt C, Fleischer H, Winkler EC. Do patients and research subjects have a right to receive their genomic raw data? An ethical and legal analysis. BMC Med Ethics 2020;21(1):7.

33. Allen J. Photoplethysmography and its application in clinical physiological measurement. Physiol Meas 2007;28(3):R1–39.

34. Lopez Perales CR, Van Spall HGC, Maeda S, et al. Mobile health applications for the detection of atrial fibrillation: a systematic review. Europace 2020;12. https://doi.org/10.1093/europace/euaa139.

35. Giebel GD, Gissel C. Accuracy of mHealth devices for atrial fibrillation screening: systematic review. JMIR Mhealth Uhealth 2019;7(6):e13641.

36. Turchioe MR, Jimenez V, Isaac S, et al. Review of mobile applications for the detection and management of atrial fibrillation. Heart Rhythm O2 2020; 1(1):35–43.

37. Pew. Mobile fact Sheet. Internet and technology. 2019. Available at: http://www.pewinternet.org/fact-sheet/mobile/#. Accessed December 7, 2020.

38. Taylor K, Silver L. Smartphone ownership is growing rapidly around the world, but not always equally, vol. 5. Pew Research Center; 2019.

39. Turakhia MP, Desai M, Hedlin H, et al. Rationale and design of a large-scale, app-based study to identify cardiac arrhythmias using a smartwatch: the Apple Heart Study. Am Heart J 2019;207:66–75.

40. Perez MV, Mahaffey KW, Hedlin H, et al. Large-Scale Assessment of a smartwatch to identify atrial fibrillation. N Engl J Med 2019;381(20):1909–17.

41. FDA. AliveCor heart monitor. 2017. Available at: https://www.accessdata.fda.gov/scripts/cdrh/cfdocs/cfPMN/pmn.cfm?ID=K142743. Accessed December 9, 2020.

42. Wegner FK, Kochhäuser S, Ellermann C, et al. Prospective blinded evaluation of the smartphone-based AliveCor Kardia ECG monitor for atrial fibrillation detection: the PEAK-AF study. Eur J Intern Med 2020; 73:72–5.

43. Haberman ZC, Jahn RT, Bose R, et al. Wireless smartphone ECG enables large-scale screening in diverse populations. J Cardiovasc Electrophysiol 2015;26(5):520–6.

44. Hickey KT, Hauser NR, Valente LE, et al. A single-center randomized, controlled trial investigating the efficacy of a mHealth ECG technology intervention to improve the detection of atrial fibrillation: the iHEART study protocol. BMC Cardiovasc Disord 2016;16:152.

45. Seto E, Ross H, Tibbles A, et al. A mobile phone–based telemonitoring program for heart failure patients after an incidence of acute decompensation (Medly-AID): protocol for a randomized controlled trial. JMIR Res Protoc 2020;9(1):e15753.

46. Halcox JPJ, Wareham K, Cardew A, et al. Assessment of remote heart rhythm sampling using the AliveCor heart monitor to screen for atrial fibrillation: the REHEARSE-AF study. Circulation 2017; 136(19):1784–94.

47. Deering TF, Hindricks G, Marrouche NF. Digital health: present conundrum, future hope or hype? Heart Rhythm 2019;16(9):1303–4.

48. Wang H. What do we know about the future? The digital health era. AHA: the early career voice. Available at: https://earlycareervoice.professional.heart.org/what-do-we-know-about-the-future-the-digital-health-era/. Accessed November 15, 2020.

49. USC center for body computing. Available at: https://www.uscbodycomputing.org/home. Accessed December 10, 2020.

50. Masterson Creber RM, Grossman LV, Ryan B, et al. Engaging hospitalized patients with personalized health information: a randomized trial of an inpatient portal. J Am Med Inform Assoc 2018;26(2): 115–23.

51. Grossman LV, Masterson Creber RM, Benda NC, et al. Interventions to increase patient portal use in vulnerable populations: a systematic review. J Am Med Inform Assoc 2019;26(8–9):855–70.

52. Caligtan CA, Carroll DL, Hurley AC, et al. Bedside information technology to support patient-centered care. Int J Med Inf 2012;81(7):442–51.

53. Prey JE, Restaino S, Vawdrey DK. Providing hospital patients with access to their medical records. AMIA annual symposium proceedings, Vol. 2014. American Medical Informatics Association; 2014. p. 1884.

54. Vawdrey DK, Wilcox LG, Collins SA, et al. A tablet computer application for patients to participate in their hospital care. AMIA Annu Symp Proc 2011; 2011:1428–35.

55. Kelly MM, Hoonakker PLT, Dean SM. Using an inpatient portal to engage families in pediatric hospital care. J Am Med Inform Assoc 2017;24(1): 153–61.

56. Larson CO, Nelson EC, Gustafson D, et al. The relationship between meeting patients' information needs and their satisfaction with hospital care and general health status outcomes. Int J Qual Health Care 1996;8(5):447–56.

57. Skeels M, Tan DS. Identifying opportunities for inpatient-centric technology. Proceedings of the 1st ACM International Health. 2010. Available at: https://dl.acm.org/doi/abs/10.1145/1882992.1883087?casa_token=QQfUd7yspRIAAAAA:9WpzYxB9sskNUTnPGvghuYubUCEeN3D6ZWlMloRZkzKNZwtGQxlLpz1kfU49vpPKKV2GpvvJp5hp. Accessed December 11, 2020.

58. Grossman LV, Choi SW, Collins S, et al. Implementation of acute care patient portals: recommendations on utility and use from six early adopters. J Am Med Inform Assoc 2018;25(4):370–9.

59. O'Leary KJ, Lohman ME, Culver E, et al. The effect of tablet computers with a mobile patient portal application on hospitalized patients' knowledge and activation. J Am Med Inform Assoc 2016;23(1):159–65.

60. Verbrugge FH, Proesmans T, Vijgen J, et al. Atrial fibrillation screening with photo-plethysmography through a smartphone camera. Europace 2019; 21(8):1167–75.

61. Väliaho E-S, Kuoppa P, Lipponen JA, et al. Wrist band photoplethysmography in detection of individual pulses in atrial fibrillation and algorithm-based detection of atrial fibrillation. Europace 2019;21(7):1031–8.

62. Guo Y, Wang H, Zhang H, et al. Mobile photoplethysmographic technology to detect atrial fibrillation. J Am Coll Cardiol 2019;74(19):2365–75.

63. Chan P-H, Wong C-K, Poh YC, et al. Diagnostic performance of a smartphone-based photoplethysmographic application for atrial fibrillation screening in a primary care setting. J Am Heart Assoc 2016;5(7). https://doi.org/10.1161/JAHA.116.003428.

64. Poh M-Z, Poh YC, Chan P-H, et al. Diagnostic assessment of a deep learning system for detecting atrial fibrillation in pulse waveforms. Heart 2018;104(23):1921–8.

65. Verma A, Champagne J, Sapp J, et al. Discerning the incidence of symptomatic and asymptomatic episodes of atrial fibrillation before and after catheter ablation (DISCERN AF): a prospective, multicenter study. JAMA Intern Med 2013;173(2):149–56.

66. Simantirakis EN, Papakonstantinou PE, Chlouverakis GI, et al. Asymptomatic versus symptomatic episodes in patients with paroxysmal atrial fibrillation via long-term monitoring with implantable loop recorders. Int J Cardiol 2017;231:125–30.

67. Heidt ST, Kratz A, Najarian K, et al. Symptoms in atrial fibrillation: a contemporary review and future directions. J Atr Fibrillation 2016;9(1):1422.

68. Reading M, Baik D, Beauchemin M, et al. Factors influencing sustained engagement with ECG self-monitoring: perspectives from patients and health care providers. Appl Clin Inform 2018;9(4):772–81.

69. Sepucha KR, Scholl I. Measuring shared decision making. Circ Cardiovasc Qual Outcomes 2014. https://doi.org/10.1161/CIRCOUTCOMES.113.000350.

70. Stacey D, Légaré F, Lewis K, et al. Decision aids for people facing health treatment or screening decisions. Cochrane Database Syst Rev 2017;4:CD001431.

71. Siebenhofer A, Ulrich L-R, Mergenthal K, et al. Primary care management for patients receiving long-term antithrombotic treatment: a cluster-randomized controlled trial. PLoS One 2019; 14(1):e0209366.

72. Zeballos-Palacios CL, Hargraves IG, Noseworthy PA, et al. Developing a conversation aid to support shared decision making: reflections on designing anticoagulation choice. Mayo Clin Proc 2019;94(4):686–96.

73. Man-Son-Hing M, Gage BF, Montgomery AA, et al. Preference-based antithrombotic therapy in atrial fibrillation: implications for clinical decision making. Med Decis Making 2005;25(5):548–59.

74. Thomson R, Parkin D, Eccles M, et al. Decision analysis and guidelines for anticoagulant therapy to prevent stroke in patients with atrial fibrillation. Lancet 2000;355(9208):956–62.

75. Thomson R, Robinson A, Greenaway J, et al, DARTS Team. Development and description of a decision analysis based decision support tool for stroke prevention in atrial fibrillation. Qual Saf Health Care 2002;11(1):25–31.

76. Durand M-A, Yen RW, O'Malley J, et al. Graph literacy matters: examining the association between graph literacy, health literacy, and numeracy in a Medicaid eligible population. PLoS One 2020; 15(11):e0241844.

77. Galesic M, Garcia-Retamero R. Graph literacy: a cross-cultural comparison. Med Decis Making 2011;31(3):444–57.

78. Turchioe MR, Myers A, Isaac S, et al. A systematic review of patient-facing visualizations of personal health data. Appl Clin Inform 2019;10(4):751.

79. Grossman LV, Feiner SK, Mitchell EG, et al. Leveraging patient-reported outcomes using data visualization. Appl Clin Inform 2018;9(3):565–75.

80. Woods SS, Evans NC, Frisbee KL. Integrating patient voices into health information for self-care and patient-clinician partnerships: veterans Affairs design recommendations for patient-generated data applications. J Am Med Inform Assoc 2016; 23(3):491–5.

81. Arcia A, Velez M, Bakken S. Style guide: an interdisciplinary communication tool to support the process of generating tailored infographics from electronic health data using EnTICE3. EGEMS (Wash DC) 2015;3(1):1120.

82. Chen C. Information visualization. Inf Visualization. 2002;1(1):1–4.

83. Mamykina L, Heitkemper EM, Smaldone AM, et al. Structured scaffolding for reflection and problem solving in diabetes self-management: qualitative study of mobile diabetes detective. J Am Med Inform Assoc 2016;23(1):129–36.

84. Garcia-Retamero R, Cokely ET. Designing visual aids that promote risk literacy: a systematic review of health research and evidence-based design heuristics. Hum Factors 2017;59(4):582–627.

85. Rudin RS, Bates DW, MacRae C. Accelerating innovation in health IT. N Engl J Med 2016;375(9):815–7.

86. Veinot TC, Mitchell H, Ancker JS. Good intentions are not enough: how informatics interventions can worsen inequality. J Am Med Inform Assoc 2018;25(8):1080–8.

87. Irizarry T, Dabbs AD, Curran CR. Patient portals and patient engagement: a state of the science review. J Med Internet Res 2015;17(6):e148.

88. Lorenc T, Petticrew M, Welch V, et al. What types of interventions generate inequalities? evidence from systematic reviews: table 1. J Epidemiol Commun Health 2013;67(2):190–3.

89. Hart JT. The inverse care law. The Lancet 1971; 297(7696):405–12.

90. Reading Turchioe M, Grossman LV, Myers AC, et al. Visual analogies, not graphs, increase patients' comprehension of changes in their health status. J Am Med Inform Assoc 2020. https://doi.org/10.1093/jamia/ocz217.

91. Toscos T, Coupe A, Wagner S, et al. Engaging patients in atrial fibrillation management via digital health technology: the impact of tailored messaging. J Innov Card Rhythm Management 2020;11(8):4209–17.

92. Mirro M, Daley C, Wagner S, et al. Delivering remote monitoring data to patients with implantable cardioverter-defibrillators: does medium matter? Pacing Clin Electrophysiol 2018;41(11):1526–35.

93. Mirro MJ, Ghahari RR, Ahmed R, et al. A patient-centered approach towards designing a novel CIED remote monitoring report. J Card Fail 2018;24(8):S77.

94. Ahmed R, Toscos T, Rohani Ghahari R, et al. Visualization of cardiac implantable electronic device data for older adults using participatory design. Appl Clin Inform 2019;10(4):707–18.

95. Baumgartner C, Fan D, Fang MC, et al. Anxiety, depression, and adverse clinical outcomes in patients with atrial fibrillation starting Warfarin: cardiovascular research network WAVE study. J Am Heart Assoc 2018;7(8). https://doi.org/10.1161/JAHA.117.007814.

96. Koleck TA, Mitha SA, Biviano A, et al. Exploring depressive symptoms and anxiety among patients with atrial fibrillation and/or flutter at the time of cardioversion or ablation. J Cardiovasc Nurs 2020. https://doi.org/10.1097/JCN.0000000000000723.

97. Chung AE, Basch EM. Potential and challenges of patient-generated health data for high-quality cancer care. JOP 2015;11(3):195–7.

98. Lobelo F, Kelli HM, Tejedor SC, et al. The Wild Wild west: a Framework to integrate mHealth Software applications and wearables to support physical activity assessment, Counseling and interventions for cardiovascular disease risk reduction. Prog Cardiovasc Dis 2016;58(6):584–94.

99. Coa K, Patrick H. Baseline motivation type as a predictor of Dropout in a healthy eating text messaging program. JMIR Mhealth Uhealth 2016; 4(3):e114.

100. Glasgow RE, Christiansen SM, Kurz D, et al. Engagement in a diabetes self-management website: usage patterns and generalizability of program use. J Med Internet Res 2011;13(1):e9.

101. Mattila E, Orsama AL, Ahtinen A, et al. Personal health technologies in employee health promotion: usage activity, usefulness, and health-related outcomes in a 1-year randomized controlled trial. JMIR Mhealth Uhealth 2013;1(2):e16.

102. King AC, Hekler EB, Grieco LA, et al. Harnessing different motivational frames via mobile phones to promote daily physical activity and reduce sedentary behavior in aging adults. PLoS One 2013;8(4):e62613.

103. Shimada SL, Allison JJ, Rosen AK, et al. Sustained use of patient portal features and Improvements in diabetes physiological measures. J Med Internet Res 2016;18(7):e179.

104. Muessig KE, Baltierra NB, Pike EC, et al. Achieving HIV risk reduction through HealthMpowerment.org, a user-driven eHealth intervention for young Black men who have sex with men and transgender women who have sex with men. Digit Cult Educ 2014;6(3):164–82.

105. Pavliscsak H, Little JR, Poropatich RK, et al. Assessment of patient engagement with a mobile application among service members in transition. J Am Med Inform Assoc 2016;23(1):110–8.

106. Horvath KJ, Alemu D, Danh T, et al. Creating effective mobile phone apps to optimize antiretroviral therapy adherence: perspectives from stimulant-using HIV-positive men who have sex with men. JMIR Mhealth Uhealth 2016;4(2):e48.

107. Miyamoto SW, Henderson S, Young HM, et al. Tracking health data is not enough: a qualitative exploration of the role of healthcare partnerships and mHealth technology to promote physical activity and to sustain behavior change. JMIR Mhealth Uhealth 2016;4(1):e5.

108. Reading Turchioe M, Burgermaster M, Mitchell EG, et al. Adapting the stage-based model of personal informatics for low-resource communities in the context of type 2 diabetes. J Biomed Inform 2020;110:103572.

109. Turchioe MR, Heitkemper EM, Lor M, et al. Designing for engagement with self-monitoring: a user-centered approach with low-income, Latino adults with Type 2 Diabetes. Int J Med Inform 2019;130:103941.

110. Cheung CC, Kerr CR, Krahn AD. Comparing 14-day adhesive patch with 24-h Holter monitoring. Future Cardiol 2014;10(3):319–22.

111. Tung CE, Su D, Turakhia MP, et al. Diagnostic yield of extended cardiac patch monitoring in patients with stroke or TIA. Front Neurol 2014;5:266.

112. Turakhia MP, Hoang DD, Zimetbaum P, et al. Diagnostic utility of a novel leadless arrhythmia monitoring device. Am J Cardiol 2013;112(4):520–4.

Moving?

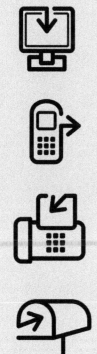

Printed and bound by CPI Group (UK) Ltd, Croydon, CR0 4YY

03/10/2024

01040367-0011